THE
SELF-CARE
SOLUTION

ALSO BY JENNIFER ASHTON, M.D., M.S.

Life After Suicide: Finding Courage, Comfort &
Community After Unthinkable Loss

Your Body Beautiful: Clockstopping Secrets to Staying
Healthy, Strong, and Sexy in Your 30s, 40s, and Beyond

Eat This, Not That! When You're Expecting:
The Doctor-Recommended Plan for Baby and You!

The Body Scoop for Girls: A Straight-Talk Guide
to a Healthy, Beautiful You

THE
SELF-CARE
SOLUTION

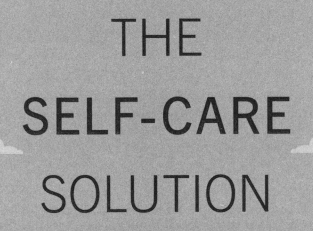

A Year of Becoming Happier, Healthier,
and Fitter—One Month at a Time

Jennifer Ashton, M.D., M.S.
with Sarah Toland

wm

WILLIAM MORROW
An Imprint of HarperCollins*Publishers*

This book is written as a source of information only. The information contained in this book should by no means be considered a substitute for the advice of the reader's qualified medical professional, who should always be consulted before beginning any new diet, exercise, or other health program.

All efforts have been made to ensure the accuracy of the information contained in this book as of the date published. The author and the publisher expressly disclaim responsibility for any adverse effects arising from the use or application of the information contained herein.

FIRST EDITION

Library of Congress Cataloging-in-Publication Data has been applied for.

ISBN 978-0-06-288542-5 (hardcover)
ISBN 978-0-06-296627-8 (international edition)

20 21 22 23 24   LSC   10 9 8 7 6 5 4 3 2 1

To self-improvers everywhere. And to my two greatest sources of inspiration and motivation, Alex and Chloe.

Contents

Introduction

I didn't set out to do a year of self-care. In fact, if you'd asked me at the start of last year if I needed to spend a year to focus on taking care of myself and my life, I probably would have told you that I didn't have time for that. Actually, I definitely would have told you that. While I've always been a self-proclaimed, relentless self-improver, the prior year had been the hardest I'd ever experienced. So when it came to self-improvement, or more important, self-care, in many respects it was the last thing on my mind.

The truth was, though, the fact that I'd kind of deprioritized self-care was perhaps the very reason why I needed it so badly. Before I embarked on this year, my emotional life had been in disarray, and taking time out to better myself seemed like the last thing I could handle. My previous year had been spent dealing with the painful aftermath of my ex-husband's suicide, and during those difficult and emotional months, the thought of taking time to focus on myself felt selfish. My kids needed me; my family needed me. To be spending time on me just felt wrong and unrealistic. I wasn't focused on the fact that hard times are often what make self-care so essential.

Perhaps that's part of the reason why I stumbled headfirst into this whole plan. It didn't start out as a plan or even a goal—it started out as one month.

As the holiday season wrapped up, I decided on a whim to give up all alcohol for January—not because I believed I was drinking too much but because I liked the idea of challenging myself to see how tweaking a regular habit could improve my life. What happened to me after one month without booze was shocking. First, I learned more about myself in thirty days than I had in years. Second, giving up alcohol for a short time dramatically changed my body, mind, mood, and attitude toward booze. Moreover, I didn't want the self-discovery and feel-good benefits I'd enjoyed by doing this experiment to end.

That month of success reinvigorated something in me. It's part of my DNA as a physician and a medical correspondent for one of the most watched television shows in America. But it's also part of who I am, Dr. Jennifer Ashton—a type A, driven, and goal-oriented human being. There's little I enjoy more than setting targets for myself and hitting them. And as a medical professional, I like using science and data to make sure I have my best chance at a bull's-eye.

And like so many people, I start every year with the hope of a New Year's resolution—often more than one. Of course, also like so many people, making resolutions stick permanently, knowing what's really beneficial to *you*, is easier said than done. But doing something for just one month? That feels achievable. That feels like the ideal length of time for experimenting. That feels like a great opportunity to understand how different kinds of self-care can have positive impacts on your life.

What emerged from that dry month was a plan, or at least the makings of one. I decided to do an experiment: each month I would tackle a different self-improvement wellness challenge, with push-ups and planks for thirty days, then meditation for thirty days, then regular aerobic exercise for thirty days, and so on, until I'd completed an entire year of minor monthly health changes. In doing so, I would understand exactly how each health improvement impacted me and become more conscious about my choices going forward.

Looking back now, I never could have guessed the profound effect that this personal experiment would have on me. From my emotional state to my diet to my sleep, I ended the year stronger than I have been in a long time. And what I learned about myself along the way was truly surprising.

While I'm a doctor and a nutritionist, it's not easy for me—or anyone, regardless of how much you take care of your body and mind—to assess what our daily habits are doing to us unless we take the time to actually examine them closely. And that's something almost nobody does. If you asked any casual observer before all this started, I likely appeared to be the epitome of near-perfect health: I was slim and fit, as I still am, and I don't smoke, use drugs, or have an alcohol problem. At that time last year, I also exercised almost daily, ate mostly whole foods, didn't suffer any mental ailments, and slept at least seven hours each night (or so I thought), while maintaining a successful career, active social life, and close family relationships.

If you're wondering why these minor changes each month produced such definitive change, the answer is simple. The impact of what we do every day for basic health—what and how much we eat and don't eat, what and how much we drink and don't drink, how much rest we get or don't get, how we move or don't move our bodies—has the potential to impact our overall health in very positive or very detrimental ways. That's because food, drink, sleep, and movement are all essential for our survival. And while these habits may have only a minor impact on our daily lives when taken in isolation, what we do and how we live each day adds up quickly, or even exponentially, when you push repeat week after week, month after month, and year after year. What this means is that if one aspect of your habits for essential health is lacking or even less than perfect, it can compound over time and end up interfering profoundly with your health and happiness, often without you knowing it.

For example, how much water you drink in one day isn't likely to send you to the hospital (although dehydration did put me in the hospital on three occasions earlier in my life, I didn't know water was to blame at the time). However, failing to consume enough water every day for weeks and months can be associated with chronic dehydration and, consequently, a whole host of physical and mental problems, including weight gain, fatigue, and bad breath.

To that end, all the health habits I focused on last year weren't inconsequential: Every monthly challenge I included in this book has been objectively linked by reams of research to being critical to overall health and happiness. They're not just arbitrary practices that affect only me; they are well-studied behaviors (or lack thereof) that can have a known and profound effect on universal wellness, no matter who you are. They are habits everyone can and should do, regardless of your age, gender, body type, fitness level, financial means, career, or lifestyle.

After a year of challenging and changing these imperative habits, I can now tell you that I'm happier and healthier than I've ever been—and not because I made a big dramatic change, went on some crazy diet, or spent three torturous months starving or working my butt off at some pricey health retreat. In short, I learned the solutions to my own self-care. And now, I want to share those solutions with you.

I used to think of self-care as mostly cosmetic—things I had to do to look better and keep up appearances, like haircuts, facials, blowouts, manicures, and spa treatments. Sure, I considered going to the gym and, more recently, meditating as part of my self-care, but I saw these habits as something to do to maintain my health, not necessarily to improve it. And also, to be honest, I looked at these things as part of my job: After all, I am the face and the voice of health and wellness for the country's number one news network. I felt I needed to look the part!

After a year of monthly health challenges, though, I now know self-care goes far beyond surface appearances and fundamental physical and mental health. Analyzing what I did with my body, mind, and free time on a daily basis forced me to realize that taking care of myself also includes how I act, think, make decisions, treat others, feel about the world, and, perhaps most important, feel about myself. Self-care now means deliberately taking the time to take care of my inner self as much as I do my outer self, giving my behaviors and emotions the same, if not more, attention than I do my hair, face, and skin.

If you're thinking, *Hey, I don't have the time to give my behaviors or emotions any attention, let alone take on any physical or mental changes,* I was in that boat last year, too. If someone had asked me to change twelve things about my daily routine, I would have balked at the idea. But now, I know that self-care isn't a matter of having time; it's a matter of readjusting what you do with that time. Self-care is also something that everyone—from the busiest CEO to the hardest working TV personality with two jobs to the person who works from home—can make time for. And as I've learned, spending just a few minutes every day to take care of yourself actually *creates* more time, because you're less stressed and more focused, energetic, and self-confident as a result. And as a mom, spending time on self-care has paid off big time in terms of what my children have learned about taking care of themselves by watching me. In fact, self-care may just be the most critical component in effective time management. If you're not doing it on a daily basis, you're likely wasting your time—and letting your health and happiness suffer as a result.

Of course, I didn't come to any of these realizations overnight because I didn't change all twelve behaviors at the same time. That's the beauty of this book; each month contains a different challenge, a new beginning, and a fresh chance for you to gain control over your health and happiness.

If you're a go-getter, you might be tempted to try to nail all twelve challenges at once. But as a doctor and a relentless self-improver, I'm here to tell you that that's exactly what you shouldn't do. As a physician, I know big dietary changes, major behavioral disruptions, and lifestyle overhauls just don't work for 99 percent of the population. I see it over and over again in my medical practice: When a patient tries to change one major thing about her diet, fitness, sleep patterns, or general routine—or she tries to change too many of these things at once—it's almost always a recipe for crash and burn. And while some patients may see temporary results from big, drastic changes, those results usually disappear in months, if not weeks or even days.

That's the biggest benefit to changing one aspect of your health, one month at a time. Improving your body and mind in bite-size pieces, over bite-size time periods, nearly guarantees lasting success. If you've ever tried a crazy fad diet, you already know this. Trying to cut gluten, dairy, meat, coffee, and alcohol all at once, for example, usually means you'll end up bingeing one night on an extra-large meat lover's pizza with a few glasses of white wine and a pint of coffee ice cream for dessert. But if you were to eliminate, let's say, only dairy, and you did it slowly over a sustained period of time while you focused on finding satisfying cheese, milk, and ice cream alternatives, you'd likely be successful. Similarly, you're more likely to sustain small changes to your regular routine than giant overhauls. And as I learned, one month's time is the perfect amount to adopt any change, then *adapt* to that change so that you can sustain it for months and continue to reap its benefits.

There's another, more scientific reason I focused on altering only one aspect of my behavior at a time. As a medical professional, I know that any good experiment can have only one independent variable—or X factor—you want to study, if you truly want to ascertain how that factor affects your body, mind, or mood. On the other hand, if you include too many variables or change too many things at once in your experiment, you won't know which variable is responsible for which effect (or lack thereof).

Go back to that example of the fad diet: If you try cutting gluten, dairy, meat, alcohol, and coffee all at once, and then your skin clears, you lose five pounds, and you suddenly have more energy, you wouldn't know which food was responsible for which result. Perhaps you're sensitive to lactose but do just fine eating gluten. Or maybe alcohol is really the culprit in your inability to lose weight, while eating too much meat is causing your skin to break out. Making small changes one at a time allows you to understand how each change impacts your health and can accurately show you the best way to sustain that change so you can truly be healthier and happier.

Let's be clear about one thing: The goal of this book and this year's journey is not necessarily to help you clear up your skin, lose five pounds, or gain more energy. While you'll likely experience all three of these results if you follow the challenges within, my goal is to teach you incredible things about your daily wellness behaviors and what you, the reader, can do to take better care of yourself.

You also don't have to complete every challenge in the exact order or way that I did. We are all unique human beings with different DNA, lives, and lifestyles, along with different practices, preferences, and physical, mental, and emotional needs. What worked for me may not work for you. Instead, what I hope to give you are the tools to let you individualize each challenge and learn the solutions to your own self-care so you can be your healthiest and happiest, too.

While I encourage you to keep an open mind and to explore each and every challenge, even those you think you may not need (Spoiler Alert: the challenges I mistakenly assumed I would ace, like September's Less Sugar Challenge, were some of my most amazing and eye-opening times), you don't have to complete every monthly challenge here. Feel free to pick and choose those that appeal to you while experimenting with other forms of self-care. For example, vegetarian or vegan readers may want to tweak May's Less Meat, More Plants Challenge to make it more about trying to eat a wider diversity of plants or less processed vegetarian and vegan foods.

When you complete a monthly challenge and start the next one, you will also be able to pick and choose those habits that you want to continue to sustain on a regular basis. After a few challenges, you'll understand how to unlock behaviors you learned in the past to access those benefits when and where you want. In other words, this book will teach you how to gain more control over your daily health and happiness.

It's important to note here that there are no mandates or expectations in this book that require you to do X or accomplish Y results in order to be successful at self-care. Just like in scientific research, you don't ever predict your results before you start an experiment. To that end, I wasn't triumphant at every monthly challenge in this book, to say the least. But during each and every challenge, I learned something invaluable about myself and, most important, what it really means to take care of me.

If I can give you one piece of advice before you start your year's journey, it's to be curious about yourself. During the last twelve months, I continually reminded myself I was doing an experiment on and for me. I remained eager to try new things and I wasn't afraid to look at my behaviors to see what did and didn't make me happy. I tried not to make assumptions or dismiss certain feelings or any results that I didn't like. After all, I wasn't trying to publish my results in a medical journal, and I didn't have to share them with my friends or family if I didn't want to. This was my year—my year to discover me and how to truly take care of my own precious self.

Similarly, this year is about you. You are the most important thing about this book, and everything you do, see, feel, and believe matters. Don't be afraid to turn the microscope around on you—it's not a serious or frightening process, especially when you examine only one little piece, one month at a time. To that end, you have nothing to lose and everything to gain.

I truly believe that everyone, no matter who you are, can live a healthier, happier, and fitter life. You have only one self, after all, one that grows and changes every day like an exquisite and intricate garden. Like a garden, you can choose to either let yourself wither and struggle to find your own light, or you can learn how to give yourself the light you need so that all your colors shine brightly, beautifully, and more boldly.

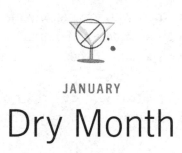

1

JANUARY

Dry Month

My Story

I don't remember the exact moment I decided to do a dry month, but it was sometime in early December of 2017. We had just finished the Thanksgiving holiday, and like most people, I was preparing for another month of work parties, holiday events, and big family dinners—all things that go hand in hand with alcohol for me and most Americans.

At the same time, I was seeing patients in my private practice, as I always do, but more often, I was having the conversation with them about their alcohol consumption. It usually went like this:

ME: How many drinks do you usually have a week?

PATIENT: Well, hmmm, I like to have a glass of wine or two a couple times a week, then maybe every Friday and Saturday, too . . . I don't know. Maybe seven?

ME: And are you having those drinks at home or out?

PATIENT: A little bit of both, I guess.

ME: Okay, so you know, one serving of wine is five ounces and one serving of liquor is one and a half ounces. But your drinks may be larger than that, especially if you're out at a restaurant or bar. Here, let me show you . . .

(Stage direction: I pull out a life-size chart of wine and cocktail glasses to show the patient just how small five ounces and one and a half ounces really is.)

ME: So, is this how much you're drinking?

PATIENT: Well . . . Probably a little more than that.

ME *(using hands to portray serving size)*: Maybe your pours are like this for wine? And maybe like this when you have a cocktail?

PATIENT: Yeah, probably.

ME: That's fine, but that means you're really having twelve or fourteen drinks a week, not seven.

PATIENT: Really?

ME: Really. And twelve to fourteen drinks per week will increase your risk of breast cancer, weight gain, obesity, depression, diabetes . . .

Yep, this was pretty much my daily script at work. I had it down pat, from the subtle pulling of the life-size cocktail chart to articulating alcohol amounts with my hands while nodding my head sympathetically.

But after years of having this conversation (and doing it well), I finally realized in December that my sympathetic nod was a little too sympathetic. I knew so intimately what these women were doing because I was doing it, too. And while I was telling them to change their habits, I was doing nothing to change my own. As they started to show more concern about the resultant increase in their risks for illnesses like breast cancer, I did, too.

I'll tell you how it started. I'm not a big drinker by any means. I drink only socially, one to two times during the workweek, and then during the weekends, if and only if I am doing something social. I also don't like ever feeling drunk. When I was in college at Columbia, I worked as a bartender three nights a week, but I never drank what we sold. Instead, I watched other people slur their words, act obnoxiously, and yell, which turned me off to drinking altogether. I was also admittedly vain and into fitness, and the idea of extra calories from alcohol seemed like a giant waste.

After college, I got married, got pregnant with my two children during medical school, then did a four-year residency in ob-gyn—there was never time to drink alcohol. That changed about five years ago, when my children were finally teenagers and able to take care of themselves, and I finally felt I had the time to enjoy a cocktail if I wanted. It started one summer, when there were lots of cook-outs and barbecues by the pool with friends, and a glass of wine just seemed like a relaxing addition to the evening. We also started having dinner at the houses of some friends who happened to be amazing cooks—and who would pour amazing wine. In the last few years, I've also become interested in wine as a hobby—learning about the grapes and tasting different varietals and vintages.

Today, I still like wine, but my preferred drink has become Casamigos Blanco tequila, served on the rocks with a slice of orange. My good friend Moll Anderson introduced it to me a few years ago as, in her words, the perfect "paleolithic drink." It contains no sugary mixers, juices, or liquors—it's basically just tequila with a slice of orange—so it's relatively low in sugar and calories.

Before January 1, 2018, I drank tequila or wine once or twice a week at special dinners or occasions, and during both nights on the weekend. Like many of my patients, I've always assumed I've stayed at or below seven drinks per week—the recommended maximum for women. But in December 2017, after having the same conversation over and over again with my patients, it suddenly dawned on me I was likely making the same mistake. I may have only been drinking seven physical glasses of alcohol per week, but like I told my patients, the serving size in one glass at any restaurant or bar was usually equivalent to much more than one and a half ounces of tequila or five ounces of wine.

The hypocrisy was a slap in the face for me: I couldn't keep doing the same routine about alcohol with my patients if I wasn't adhering to the same advice. I had to change my habits, and when I realized that in December, I figured the New Year was the perfect time to start. I don't believe in resolutions—science shows they don't work—but I do believe in challenging ourselves to change small specific actions or habits. Unlike resolutions, research has found that challenging yourself to take on a specific, actionable, and manageable change can help you sustain that change until it becomes part of your daily routine.

I had made up my mind. I was going to do a dry month. On New Year's Eve, I enjoyed a celebratory lunch with rosé and dinner with tequila, feeling no apprehension for the month ahead. I had to draw a line in the sand somewhere, and this was it.

Doctor's Notes

OVERCOMING ALCOHOLISM AND ALCOHOL DISORDERS

A dry month is a wellness challenge designed to help individuals with normal, healthy drinking habits benefit from the ramifications of giving up alcohol for thirty days. If you have a problem with or dependency on drinking, this challenge is not for you. Instead, you should speak with your physician or seek professional help. Warning signs of a problem with alcohol include suffering frequent hangovers, feeling like you need a drink or can't stop drinking after you start, making poor or dangerous decisions while drinking, and incurring negative relationship, career, or other personal consequences when you do drink. If you think you have a problem with alcohol, don't try to hide it or be embarrassed: it's common, and professional guidance can help you overhaul your life.

Week 1
Share the Secret: The Best Thing to Do When You're Tempted to Drink

On New Year's Day 2018, I was in Boston with my family for an ice hockey tournament for Chloe, my athletic daughter who is a top-scoring forward on her travel team. Unlike most holidays, this one wasn't replete with tempting eating or drinking experiences—no dinner out at a fancy restaurant or New Year's party to attend. But I still woke up that very first day and thought, *Okay, here we go. This is Day 1.*

Physically, I didn't have a desire to drink, but psychologically, I was thirsty. Blame it on something doctors like to call the deprivation effect: when you tell patients they can't eat, drink, or do something, that's all they want to eat, drink, or do—or at the very least, they fixate on eating, drinking, or doing it. So, on the first day of the month, even though I didn't physically or socially crave a drink, I kept thinking about how I wouldn't be able to have an alcoholic beverage for the entire month. *Seriously, the whole month?!*, I kept thinking.

But that psychological obsession dissipated after the first day, primarily because of a serendipitous opportunity that happened to occur right after the New Year. As the chief medical correspondent for *Good Morning America,* I was asked to do a segment the following day that would cover the kind of complications women can experience when they consume more than the recommended weekly maximum of alcohol. During the segment, which aired live on January 2, I discussed all the reasons why women shouldn't have more than seven drinks per week, then I announced to *GMA* anchor Robin Roberts that I was personally doing a dry month.

To my surprise—and to the surprise of the show's producers— the segment exploded in popularity among viewers. More than five million people watch and listen to *GMA* every morning, and I couldn't believe how many of our regular viewers were excited about the challenge. Soon after the segment aired, hundreds of comments started pouring into my social media pages, along with *GMA's*, remarks like, *I'll do it with you!* and *Great idea, count me in!*

The producers were impressed and asked me to detail the challenge in a Facebook Live following the show. That video received over three hundred thousand views in less than twenty-four hours—a remarkable response even for one of the most watched television shows in the United States. Apparently, the idea of a dry month was striking a chord with many Americans. And it appeared to me that people didn't just want to give up alcohol for a month—they wanted to participate in the challenge with others and feel part of a community.

Later that week, I met with Joanna Coles, the former editor in chief of *Cosmopolitan* and chief content officer for Hearst. Even she had seen the segment. Joanna is from England, though, where she told me the concept of drying out in January is common. I couldn't believe it. An entire country gave up alcohol in January every year? Knowing that thousands of others were making this an annual ritual made me feel like I had a whole team of supporters behind me, many who had a proven track record of success with going dry.

The first week of January, it was relatively easy for me to forget about alcohol, thanks to my normal routine. I often get up daily at five in the morning to appear on *GMA*, then see patients in my medical office in New Jersey until at least six at night. Oftentimes, I don't have the chance to exercise until the evening, so I usually head to the gym right after work. When I finally get home, I'm often too exhausted to even entertain the idea of going out for a drink.

But that first weekend, Chloe had another ice hockey game, this time at home, where all the parents often get together to tailgate beforehand. What this entails is lots of mulled cider, wine, hoagies, and snacks for some forty adults—in other words, it's a real tailgate party. My problem: I have a particular fondness for mulled cider. Here was my first temptation.

When I arrived at the tailgate party that day, I announced to the entire tent that I was doing a dry month. I felt a little silly and self-conscious about it, but I thought telling everyone right off the bat would be easier than repeatedly refusing drinks or having to make up multiple excuses or explain the Dry Challenge over and over again. I also hoped that telling people, whether parents I knew or total strangers, would hold me accountable—and I was right. Nobody offered me a drink and I wasn't tempted to take one.

After the game, my brother and his family joined us for lunch at one of our favorite Italian restaurants. Every time I go to this restaurant, I order a glass of wine—it just complements the food so beautifully. But I didn't want to be tempted this time, so after what I learned at the tailgate, I announced to my family after we sat down that I was doing a dry month. My brother, the perennial jokester, responded that he was doing a wet month, trying to drink more than he usually did. This added levity to the exchange, and even though he and others at the table ordered wine, it didn't bother me at all.

During that lunch, I had an interesting revelation. I'd been to this restaurant many times before, but when I was here without wine, I found myself paying closer attention to what I ordered. There was no alcohol to distract me from making healthy food choices or to lower my inhibitions so I didn't care if I had another slice of garlic bread. And since I was getting no pleasure from the wine I wasn't drinking, I discovered that I was focused more on enjoying my food. At the end of the meal, I thought I'd even eaten less since I felt more satisfied with what I'd already consumed.

Week 2
If You Don't Want to Stop Drinking for Your Health, Do It for Your Skin

On January 8, I woke up to a lovely surprise: my skin looked totally different. I've always had a case of mild rosacea, or small red bumps on my face, but when I looked in the mirror that morning, my face looked significantly less ruddy. My skin also looked like it had more elasticity and was even plumper—both results of better hydration. I even felt like I saw slightly fewer wrinkles around my eyes and mouth.

Working in television on-air every day, I'm highly attuned to the health of my skin. TV makeup is harsh and is always caked on thickly, requiring what seems to amount to a sandblaster to remove. I try to take off my makeup as soon as I'm off-air and certainly before I go to bed at night. So, when I wake up, my morning face is the most virginal form of my skin I'll see all day. I like to take stock of what I look like then, and I was surprised to see such a remarkable difference in one week's time.

I put on my doctor's cap and thought about this: the only variable I had changed in my routine of late was not drinking. I knew alcohol was dehydrating and had heard from dermatologists it was detrimental to skin, but I had never believed giving up booze would have this kind of effect. The impact was even greater given we were in the middle of winter, when my skin usually looks its worst due to cold, dry air outdoors and dehydrating indoor heat.

When I showed up at *GMA* that morning, I asked my makeup artist, Lisa, if my skin transformation was only in my head or if she noticed a difference, too. When she told me my skin looked younger, healthier, and more hydrated, I felt like someone had spiked my coffee, I was so giddy with glee. This no-drinking thing was paying off in ways I didn't imagine.

During the second week, I also noticed that avoiding alcohol wasn't as socially or logistically difficult as I thought it would be. I didn't feel as if I were depriving myself or staring at the calendar, counting down the days until I could have a tequila or a glass of wine. I attributed this to the fact I knew many other people were doing it with me—not only half of Great Britain but hundreds of my followers on social media as well, along with *GMA* viewers. It felt as though I was running a marathon with thousands of other people who would be disappointed if I dropped out at mile 12. And

I didn't want to drop out: the challenge aspect of the month made it fun, the support made it easy, and the benefits I was now seeing so quickly made it all the more worthwhile.

Week 3
A Surprising Way to Make Going Without Alcohol More Enjoyable

On January 17, past the month's halfway mark, I was out to dinner with a friend, sitting at the bar, and she ordered prosecco while I ordered what had become my new social standard: a glass of sparkling water in a wineglass, which still felt like a sophisticated drink, albeit alcohol-free. I had been to bars many times since the beginning of the month, so sitting at one without drinking was hardly a new experience, but when the bartender set my friend's prosecco in front of me, I picked it up and put it to my lips.

Thankfully, I had told my friend, like everyone else I knew, that I was doing a dry month, and she squealed when she saw me poised with her prosecco in hand. It had just been muscle memory—I simply forgot for a split second about the challenge. I thanked her and passed her the glass, without a single pang of envy—I was happy to have my water and stay focused on chatting with my friend. Without alcohol, I had noticed this was much easier; that is, the company of friends and family was much more enjoyable without drinking. Not only was I never distracted by the decision of whether to have a second drink or what to order if I did, but moreover, I simply wasn't distracted by the booze at all and those feelings when we drink of being a little foggy and less focused.

At the end of the week, my skin looked even better, less red and dry than the week before, while my skin tone also appeared as if it had improved. I wasn't dealing with any breakouts or patches of troubled skin—in fact, I felt like I was glowing and that I could get away with wearing less makeup. Better still, my stomach felt flatter, and my little belly paunch or mommy pouch that I can't stand had seriously receded.

After this development, I started to think about it. If my skin looked better, my belly was flatter, and I was enjoying my food and company more without alcohol, why did I choose to drink in the first place? Is it an automatic decision to do what friends or family at a restaurant or party or at someone's home for dinner do? Or did I really just love the taste of wine and tequila? Since I stick to just one or two drinks at a time, booze's physical effects on me were minor at best. So what about this social custom did I enjoy? I began to think that, going forward, drinking needed to be more of a conscious decision for me rather than an automatic reaction in social situations.

Week 4
How Going Dry Changed How I'll Look at Alcohol Forever

After these realizations, the last week was surprisingly easy—so easy, in fact, that I had already decided that I was going to moderate my drinking for the rest of the year. What I was going to do, I vowed, was record all the times I drank during the week on my wall calendar and then track my weekly "balance" of drinks just like I did with my bank account. I would count each drink as two actual servings and make sure I never exceeded seven servings per week.

After three consistent weeks of avoiding all alcohol, I noticed another change during Week 4: I had more energy—which is saying something considerable, since I'm already a high-energy person. Moreover, I truly believed I looked better, which could have something to do with the fact that I had a more positive outlook without alcohol, but I also knew I was more hydrated and getting deeper sleep than I had been in months, which was affecting both my skin and my waistline.

The ramifications were also psychological: I was proud of myself. Before the month began, I had wanted to see if I could challenge myself to conquer a small lifestyle change that seemed difficult, and I'd succeeded with more ease and enjoyment than I had ever imagined.

Going dry for thirty days, which is how long some experts say we need to change a habit, was affecting my aptitude and desire to drink. I knew after the challenge ended that I wanted to change the way I interacted with alcohol. And I had a simple plan to achieve that very sustainable goal of no more than seven drinks per week by writing down all my weekly cocktails and counting each tumbler or glass as two servings.

The last day of the month, instead of dreaming about my first blanco tequila or pinot noir, I felt so charged by the physical and mental benefits of not drinking that I decided to extend my dry month into the first week of February. After that, I was headed to the Caribbean on vacation, so I figured it would be a nice way to wrap up my dry spell by enjoying my first drink back somewhere truly warm and relaxing. But to be honest, I now don't even remember having that first drink on vacation—it wasn't a major moment or paramount synapsis of pleasure, even after five weeks sober. Looking back on it now, this fact further corroborated the realization that I was just drinking out of mere social habit, not necessarily because I enjoyed it so much.

There was another reason I wanted to continue my dry month— and it had nothing to do with not drinking per se. Instead, I was hooked on the idea and practice of challenging myself to be healthier. The month had not only improved my physical and mental outlook in unforeseen ways, it had also been psychologically rewarding, emotionally fulfilling, and personally fun. I liked the science-experiment aspect of the month: How would I do this? What could I learn about myself? What could I learn about others?

More so, what helped me enjoy the challenge were the hundreds of tweets, Facebook posts, and Instagram comments from viewers, followers, and friends alike. People were motivated by the idea of a challenge and excited to join me—you would have thought I was offering a month of free candy, not the chance to avoid alcohol. The response had increased my sense of achievement, and I didn't want to lose this amazing community support group I had helped form. So why not keep it together with another challenge for February . . . and beyond?

JANUARY DRY MONTH:
The Science Behind Giving Up Alcohol

Like all monthly challenges in this book, I chose going dry because it's a small lifestyle change that has been shown by scientific research to have big benefits to your physical, emotional, and mental health. How much potential a dry month has to change your personal health depends on how much you drink—for example, if you have only one glass of wine every few weeks, going dry won't have a drastic impact on your wellness profile. But if you're like most Americans, giving up alcohol for thirty days can have significant and lasting effects. Many of these health benefits you may already know, but here are some more surprising ways giving up booze for thirty days can overhaul your health.

You Definitely May Drink More Than You Think

Most people drink more than they realize. According to recent research published in the journal *Addiction,* people who would be low-risk drinkers—that is, women and men who consume fewer than ten and fifteen drinks per week, respectively—underreport how much alcohol they have by an incredible 76 percent, effectively accounting for only one of four drinks they enjoy.

The reasons are complex. First, we don't always remember how many drinks we have, as we often consume them during active social situations—and logging our weekly alcohol intake isn't exactly a top priority for most people. It's also difficult, psychologists say, to be truly honest with ourselves about our alcohol consumption, similar to the way many of us would rather forget how much junk food or candy we eat: keeping a mental track is simply a reminder we're doing something detrimental to our bodies, a fact we don't necessarily want to face.

But numerous studies show we're also drinking more because we're being served more—and that's whether we make our own drinks or they're poured for us by bartenders or waitstaff. Here's how it works. In the United States, a standard drink is considered to be anything that contains fourteen grams of pure alcohol, which is equivalent to twelve ounces of beer, five ounces of wine, or one and a half ounces of liquor, including vodka, gin, rum, whiskey, and tequila.

But multiple studies show alcoholic beverages served at bars and restaurants, along with those we make ourselves, usually contain more booze than fourteen grams—or more than the respective ounces for beer, wine, and liquor that this number indicates. For example, one 2008 investigation published in *Alcoholism: Clinical and Experimental Research* uncovered that wine poured at restaurants contains, on average, 43 percent more volume than the standard five ounces, while mixed drinks contain 42 percent more volume and draft beers 22 percent more volume.

You're even more likely to be overserved if you're pouring wine, beer, or cocktails at home. Not only do Americans underestimate realistic servings of food and drink in our modern age of supersized everything, our glassware may also be to blame. According to a 2017 study from researchers at the University of Cambridge, the average size of a wineglass has grown sevenfold in the last three hundred years so that now most glasses can hold 15 ounces of alcohol. Even if you poured yourself a half glass, that's still 7.5 ounces—equivalent to a serving and a half of wine.

Want to know if you're pouring supersize drinks at home? Try using a measuring cup or single shot glass to measure out five ounces of wine, twelve ounces of beer, or one and a half ounces of liquor, pouring that amount in the glassware you typically use. You might be surprised by how abnormally small the amount looks to what you normally pour.

Just One Drink per Day Can Raise Your Breast Cancer Risk

One in eight American women will be diagnosed with breast cancer at some point in her lifetime. That's a big percentage, so it's not surprising that many of my patients are panicked about developing the disease.

One of the most common questions I get in my practice is about birth control pills—whether the medication increases a patient's risk of breast cancer and if she should stop taking the drug because of it. What I tell women is that the science on birth control pills and cancer is not cut-and-dried. Some studies show a small increased risk of breast cancer, but not in the number of breast cancer deaths. On the other hand, other studies show a marked reduction in the risks of ovarian and uterine cancer among women who take or have taken birth control pills.

While the data on breast cancer and the pill may be cloudy, the research on alcohol isn't: having just one alcoholic drink per day increases breast cancer risk. Still, I've not had one patient say she'd like to give up alcohol altogether to reduce her risk. And I get that: it's easier mentally and from a lifestyle perspective to stop taking a pill and use other contraceptive forms than it is to give up a popular, widespread social habit.

So how does alcohol boost breast cancer risk? For starters, scientists believe alcohol raises levels of estrogen and other hormones in a woman's body that can contribute to the disease. Booze is also a great source of empty calories, which, as you likely know, can quickly turn into excess weight, which is associated with an increased risk of cancer of all kinds. Finally, alcohol has also been shown to lower the body's ability to absorb folate and even damage DNA, both of which can impact breast cancer risk.

For these reasons, most doctors advise that women who have an elevated risk of breast cancer due to family history or other lifestyle factors avoid alcohol altogether or cut back significantly, meaning no more than two drinks per week. According to the American Cancer Society, women without a high risk should drink no more than one serving of alcohol per week.

Don't Believe Everything You Read About Alcohol Being Good for Your Heart

Breast cancer isn't the only chronic disease linked to alcohol intake. According to the American Cancer Society, booze has been shown to increase the risk of cancer for the liver, colon, rectum, mouth, throat, esophagus, and larynx. The more you drink, the greater your cancer risk, researchers say.

Some of you may be thinking, *Isn't alcohol good for your heart?* And yes, studies do show that drinking in moderation, meaning no more than one drink per day for women and two drinks daily for men, can have a positive effect on heart health by reducing the risk of blood clots and raising "good" HDL cholesterol.

But drinking more than a moderate weekly amount of alcohol can hurt your heart by boosting blood pressure and contributing to obesity, both of which raise the risk of heart disease, heart failure, and stroke. A 2017 University of Cambridge study also found that consuming more than five drinks per week raises the risk of stroke, fatal aneurysm, heart failure, and death.

Alcohol Wreaks Havoc on Your Sleep

Drinking can have the effect of a strong cup of coffee when it comes to how much and well we sleep. Why? Well, if you've had just one drink in your lifetime, you know alcohol is a relaxant that has a calming effect—it's why many people rely on a glass of wine or whiskey to help fall asleep. It works, too: alcohol boosts the body's production of the sleep-inducing chemical adenosine, but the effect is only temporary. When this production ends and the adenosine wears off, the result is a big jolt in your circadian rhythm, or your body's internal clock, causing you suddenly to feel more awake.

That's not all, either. Alcohol has also been shown to block REM sleep, the most restorative type our bodies need for overall health. The less REM you get, the more likely you'll also wake up groggy the next day. Finally, drinking can worsen breathing problems like snoring and sleep apnea and interfere with your wake-sleep cycle by causing you to get up more often to use the bathroom.

Drinking Can Make You Gain Weight in Sneakier Ways Than You Know About

While this shouldn't be a shocker, I'm still surprised by the number of patients who don't know or want to admit that alcohol—and not necessarily the bread, pasta, or other carbs they consume—is preventing them from losing the weight they want. When you drink alcohol, your body quickly converts booze's simple carbs into sugar because there's no fat, protein, or fiber to slow that conversion down. This makes every alcoholic beverage you drink akin to consuming sugar packets. And if you prefer cocktails with sugary ingredients like soda, juice, or simple syrup, you're adding even more empty calories to your boozy intake.

Five ounces of wine contains approximately 120 calories—and you're likely drinking more than five ounces in one glass, as research shows. That means that drinking one glass of wine daily gives you 850 extra calories per week and nearly 3,500 extra calories per month—the equivalent of one pound of fat. Drink more than one glass per day or add sugary ingredients to a cocktail and that caloric intake will climb steadily.

Alcohol also lowers your inhibitions, including your resolve to order healthy grilled salmon instead of fattening nachos. When you drink, you're also less likely to pay attention to how much you're eating. I know that if I order a margarita at a Mexican restaurant, it's pretty much hardwired in my brain to eat chips while I sip. There's a psychological and social connection between consuming food and alcohol, and breaking that association can be difficult while continuing to drink.

Booze Can Make Your Skin Look Bad

You don't need science to tell you that drinking dehydrates your body. But we could all use a reminder on just how bad booze is for our skin. To start, alcohol interferes with liver function and the organ's ability to detoxify cells, including skin cells. That's why patients with liver problems often have skin problems, too, like yellow tone, enlarged pores, increased dryness, breakouts, and sagging.

Alcohol also triggers systemic inflammation in the body, causing our skin cells and blood vessels to flare up—one reason our faces turn red when we drink. Consume enough alcohol over time, though, and you can stretch those blood vessels and break capillaries in your face, causing that redness to become a permanent fixture. Too much alcohol can also interfere with your body's ability to absorb vitamin A, which helps produce the collagen that keeps skin plump and elastic.

Alcohol Messes with Your Moods

While having a cocktail with friends can make you feel momentarily better about life, there's no two ways about it: alcohol is a depressant and will increase the risk of depression, anxiety, and other mood disorders, no matter how much or little you drink. Ever wake up after a big night out and feel despondent about life? That's likely the effect of too much alcohol. Those who drink heavily have a higher risk of self-harm, suicide, and psychosis.

Drinking Can Drain Your Bank Account

This detriment may not be scientific per se, but one of the many benefits of a dry month is that you'll save—and a significant amount if you primarily drink at bars or restaurants, where prices are marked up considerably.

At the end of the month, I calculated that I'd saved at least $300 by not drinking for thirty days. That's the equivalent of a nice new pair of shoes (or several pairs of shoes on sale). Multiply this by twelve and I'd save $3,600 per year if I didn't drink. Consider that a European vacation, a down payment on a new car, or a kitchen redesign.

JANUARY DRY MONTH: Your Story

From a health and wellness standpoint, doing a dry month is a no-brainer. And while it was relatively easy for me, giving up booze isn't a cinch for everyone, especially if alcohol is an integral part of your social or work life, or you rely on it to relax and de-stress. Here are ten ways to make the Dry Challenge easier and more sustainable.

1. TELL EVERYONE YOU KNOW YOU'RE DOING A DRY MONTH. This is my number one tip to have a successful month. Announcing that I was doing a dry month to everyone I knew and met, whether a single friend or a full party, nearly guaranteed my sobriety in several ways. First, no one will

ask you if you want a drink or hand you champagne or a cocktail after you tell them you're not drinking. This also alleviates any peer pressure: there's nothing wrong with you and you're not a prude or no fun, you're just not drinking for January.

Telling everyone also makes you accountable for your actions. After all, you'll look fairly silly and capricious if you suddenly order a mojito or ask for wine after announcing your intent to stay sober for a month to an entire party, at the dinner table, or even to a single friend.

While you may feel self-conscious announcing something so personal or sharing your resolution before anyone even asks, don't. I found that 99 percent of the people I told I was doing a dry month not only responded positively but even told me that they admired my resolve and wished they could do it, too. And remember, this is January, a month when many people make resolutions, so chances are you aren't the only one in the room who's trying to stick with a goal, whether that's weight loss, getting to the gym, or eating healthier.

2. USE SOCIAL MEDIA TO CREATE A SUPPORT NETWORK. I can't underestimate the power that social media had on helping me stay dry. The hundreds of comments and tweets made me feel like I had a whole league of supporters rooting for me and strengthened my resolve to stay sober, not just for myself but for my entire team, too. You don't need a zillion comments, retweets, or shares—even just one friend who likes a post or comments with encouragement can motivate you when you feel like giving up. Finally, almost everyone uses Facebook, Twitter, and Instagram to trumpet their successes—when they finish a race, cook an amazing meal, or find a new job. By doing the same about your dry month, you're turning the challenge into something to be admired and celebrated.

3. SUGGEST ACTIVITIES THAT HAVE NO ASSOCIATION WITH AL-
    COHOL. Here's one thing I know: no matter who you are,
    you don't need alcohol to have a good time. Remember how
    much fun you had as a kid going outside, playing games
    with your friends, doing sports, and going to parties? There's
    no reason you can't do all the same things now—and enjoy
    them just as much—without alcohol.

    Some social activities I like to do that don't include drink-
    ing are trying new exercise classes with friends, visiting a
    new coffee shop, and seeing a new exhibit at a museum or
    gallery. I also like going for long walks with friends, organiz-
    ing a girls' night with a fun movie or Netflix show, taking
    cooking classes, and going shopping. There are a million
    ways to enjoy friends and family without alcohol as soon as
    you start thinking outside bars and restaurants.

4. AT BARS OR RESTAURANTS, ORDER AN ALCOHOL-FREE DRINK
    IN A COCKTAIL OR WINEGLASS. I got this tip from a *GMA*
    viewer who tweeted that he felt less tempted to drink at bars
    or restaurants if he ordered a seltzer water in a wineglass—
    giving the same sensation of a sophisticated adult drink, but
    without the booze. If you prefer cocktails, try seltzer water
    with a twist in a tumbler or even a martini glass—this also
    looks like a cocktail, doubling as a good subterfuge if you
    don't want people to ask why you're not drinking. Finally,
    many bars now offer a bevy of mocktails—alcohol-free cock-
    tails that taste and look like the real thing. Just be careful
    about the calories: many are made from the same sugary in-
    gredients in cocktails. If you can, opt for alcohol-free drinks
    that include soda water, seltzer, kombucha, fresh fruit, tea,
    and/or vegetable juices.

5. TURN THE GYM INTO YOUR HAPPY HOUR. One reason I wasn't
    tempted to meet friends at bars after work is that I went to the

gym instead. Once there, I saw plenty of people I knew—my gym friends—which makes it feel similar to a social outing, or certainly more social than going home. What's more, an hour lifting heavy weights or spinning to loud music at a SoulCycle class provides a far more effective form of stress relief than any tequila, no matter the vintage. After the gym, the idea of going out was the last thing I wanted to do: I already had plenty of serotonin surging through my brain thanks to the exercise, and the idea of undoing my taxing physical work with a toxic drink wasn't appealing.

6. FIND ALTERNATIVE WAYS TO RELIEVE STRESS. If you use alcohol to relax after work, you'll need to find another way to unwind during your Dry Challenge. The good news: Relaxation is fairly easy to find if you know where and how to look. For example, research shows simply being outside, seeing green trees, parks, or the water, can have an immediate and significant calming effect. You already know exercise is a great way to purge stress, but similar activities that will get your blood pumping like dancing or sex can also do wonders. Meditation, deep breathing, and yoga are all well-known methods for reducing anxiety and promoting better mood, while studies show listening to classical music, talking with a close friend, or participating in a repetitive motion like knitting or painting can also relieve stress.

    My outlet when I'm superstressed is online shopping. I don't spend money, but find it relaxing just to look at purses, shoes, and jackets and imagine wearing all of them in various combinations. I've also been known to end a hectic day with a marathon run of *Orange Is the New Black* or *Billions*.

7. PROMISE TO TAKE A TRIP OR BUY NEW SHOES WITH THE BOOZE MONEY YOU'RE SAVING. Whenever you're tempted to trade in your seltzer for a Syrah, remember how much money you're

saving by not ordering that $10 (or $20 in New York City) glass of wine. If it helps, calculate how much you'll save if you stay dry for the entire month and promise to treat yourself to something with that money if you're successful for all four weeks. The next time you feel Syrah's siren call, visualize that gift to yourself.

8. USE THE OLD-SCHOOL CALENDAR CROSS-OFF METHOD. There's a reason why there's now a proliferation of smartphone apps that let you digitally cross off calendar days to mark your progression toward a goal or end date: it works. Being able to see your success, whether displayed on a smartphone app or on an old-school wall calendar, can be immensely motivating and rewarding. Before I started the month, I bought a wall calendar and hung it up in a visible place in my kitchen, then physically crossed off each and every day I didn't have a drink. Not only was slashing through the days with a bright pen a physically gratifying feeling so was being able to see all the days I'd been dry. After just a few days, I didn't want to break the bright-red streak and began to look forward to the end of the evening when I could mark another day down as successful.

9. THERE'S NOTHING WRONG WITH SAYING NO. Can't go to a bar or party without having a drink? My advice: stay home. There's nothing wrong with saying no—think of it instead as saying yes to yourself, your health, a better night's sleep, a trimmer waistline, and the dozens of other benefits that giving up alcohol imparts. There will be plenty more invites come February 1 and missing a few happy hours or parties for thirty days won't cause you to fall off the social calendar with family and friends. If you do end up going and having a drink, I guarantee you'll feel guiltier than you would about saying no to a bar or party invite.

10. NOT DRINKING IS LIKE HORSEBACK RIDING: IF YOU FALL OFF, THE BEST THING IS TO GET RIGHT BACK ON. Don't beat yourself up if you slip up and have a drink. Everyone makes mistakes. The bigger mistake is letting a fall off the bandwagon turn into an all-night tumble. Stop at one drink, go home (or pour it out), and get back to trying to stay dry the following day. Nobody's perfect. And if you read this whole book, you have eleven more months of lifestyle challenges to improve your game, overhaul your health, and help turn challenge into lasting change.

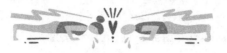

2

FEBRUARY

Push-Ups and Planks

My Story

In 2018, the year I did my January challenge, I turned forty-nine years old, which meant I'd be fifty the following year—a full half century of breathing, eating, and sleeping on this planet. I was a little apprehensive and excited at the same time.

Was I going to have a midlife crisis? Maybe, but I decided that if I did, I wanted to do something that would make me look and feel better as I age, not just jolt me into feeling alive again because I went skydiving, bought a convertible, or sold all my worldly belongings and moved to Mexico. My midlife crisis would be this book or attempting to complete a whole year of health and wellness challenges that would force me to turn my doctor's eye on my own habits and evaluate what I was doing right, what I was doing wrong, and what I could improve about my health with little lifestyle tweaks.

The word *little* is key to that last sentence—and to this challenge at large. Trying to adopt a significant lifestyle change—like a low-carb diet when you primarily eat processed carbs or a daily exercise program when you haven't worked out in years—isn't realistic or sustainable. While ambitious wellness goals are admirable and can result in tremendous benefits—and I certainly wouldn't stop anyone from trying—targeting something that's unrealistic, if not impossible, can set you up for lasting feelings of failure, causing you to dread the idea of healthy eating or exercise altogether.

What does this have to do with push-ups and planks? After I finished my dry month, I was so excited and satisfied that I'd been able to do it—and do it well—that immediately after it ended, I wanted another bite-size goal to target. Moreover, during my dry month, I had developed this incredible support group of viewers, friends, and followers on social media who had become a team of fellow challenge takers, and I didn't want to let that community go. They hadn't just been excited to go dry with me, they were giddy, and that giddiness was contagious. I was swept up in the social media outpouring, and I wanted to continue to ride the tide.

But what could I do for a February challenge? I weighed a lot of options before I decided. Since I had just done something for my general health, I wanted a mission that would specifically affect my body or fitness levels. I also wanted a challenge I could do anywhere—no gym, class, pool, or bike path necessary—and that would produce results even if I did it for only minutes, not hours, per day.

That's how I settled on the monthly challenge of push-ups and planks. About six years ago, I discovered the boutique exercise class Bar Method. During the class, you do lots of muscle-lengthening and -strengthening exercises at a ballet barre and on the floor, including push-ups and planks. There was no physical mercy when it came to these exercises, either, with participants doing at least forty-five push-ups per class and holding planks for several minutes.

After nearly two months of taking Bar Method classes four times a week, my body changed. For the first time in my life, my arms looked shredded—not just more muscular but totally toned. I couldn't believe it. I had always wanted ripped arms, but no matter how much I lifted or worked out in the gym, they remained these chicken-wing-like contraptions, maybe with no fat on them, but with no real muscle, either. But suddenly I had definition in my deltoids and triceps, and what Chloe and I like to call "caps"— graceful little rounds of muscles on top of the shoulders that look like elegant epaulettes.

Concurrently, I felt stronger throughout my core, tighter and more pulled up. While my posture has traditionally been terrible—I often slouch and my stomach pooches out if I don't consciously suck it in—I was now standing more erect, with my shoulders back, hips tucked, and stomach flat, thanks to all the planking I was doing.

I was both mystified and delighted by this transformation, and the only thing I had done differently over the past two months was push-ups and planks—the other Bar Method exercises had already been part of my regular gym routine. The experience corroborated the idea that you *can* change how you look and feel when you start doing something every day, even if it's only for several minutes at a time. As a doctor, I knew this, but to see and feel it firsthand was eye-opening.

Keeping that experience in mind, I wanted to structure February's challenge so that I would get the same arm-shredding benefits I had from Bar Method. This meant, I figured, trying to do as many push-ups and planks as I could every day for thirty consecutive days. But to make this goal attainable, I knew I had to begin the month with a relatively modest number of push-ups and not too crazy of a plank time, then attempt to increase both reps and duration as the weeks progressed.

When I announced the Push-ups and Planks Challenge on social media, people responded enthusiastically and that they were excited for a physical feat that seemed so simple and didn't require anything more than a few minutes per day. Some followers tweeted they could do only one push-up or had to do them on their knees or needed to modify the plank in order to hold it for more than a few seconds. And that's okay. The point is to try to do as many push-ups and planks as *you* can—and to get better at both exercises as the month goes on—no matter where or how you have to start.

What did I start with? I had stopped going to Bar Method classes several years ago, lured away by the temptation of trying other boutique fitness classes like SoulCycle. As a result, I had unfortunately let push-ups and planks slip from my workout routine.

I still figured, though, that I could do at least twenty-five standard push-ups and maintain good form, bringing my chest as close as possible to the floor, and I knew I could hold a plank for more than a minute if I had to. But these numbers seemed a little extreme to start with if I was going to do both daily and increase progressively. And I certainly didn't want to disappoint myself or my social media challenge team by burning out by Week 2. I decided to start the month with twenty push-ups and one forty-five-second plank. This would still be taxing on Day 1, but not impossible by Day 14 if I wanted to increase my reps and time.

Week 1
How a Ninety-Second Sweat Session Can Pump You Up (Literally)

On Day 1, while dressed in street clothes and in a hotel room in Massachusetts, I dropped to the floor and cranked out twenty push-ups, then held my plank for a full forty-five seconds, as my daughter, Chloe, watched. When I stood up, I was breathing harder than I thought I would. Even though the sequence had taken me no more than ninety seconds, I was surprised to see I wasn't coolly filing my nails afterward.

I continued to do both exercises consecutively, one after another, usually first thing in the morning, dropping down on the floor of my bedroom only after I had a cup of coffee (because I need coffee immediately to power through anything, even if I'm just sitting still). Within the first week, I had developed a routine: turn on the shower and, while the water was heating up, drop and hold the plank first, then crank out the push-ups.

That first week, I managed to nail the challenge six out of the seven days. That's great, right? I know, but I was upset over my first challenge hiccup. On that day, I went to the gym, where I lifted weights. By the time I realized I hadn't done a single plank or push-up, I was exhausted—my arms also physically hurt from lifting—and I blew it off.

Skipping a day wasn't easy for me, though. Instead, it instigated a negotiation between myself and my inner logic that went like this: Self: *Do you really need to do push-ups and planks when you'd already been to the gym for an hour?* Logic: No. Self: *But aren't you slacking on this challenge? The goal is to do them. Every. Single. Day.* Logic: Yes. Self: *Well, that's contradictory! So, what should I do?* Logic. *It's late. Do them tomorrow instead.* And that's what I did. But I do believe that missing that one day was motivation enough for me to make sure I did my push-ups and planks religiously every other day of the week.

At the end of the week, I didn't notice a difference in how I looked or felt. I had, after all, been doing push-ups and planks for only six days—not exactly the kind of effort it takes for an instant six-pack. But after that first day in the Massachusetts hotel, the exercises had become easier—or at least easier to incorporate into my morning routine—and I finished the week excited it'd been less taxing than I originally imagined. I'd also bumped up my number of push-ups by at least a rep every day, increasing my plank duration by five to ten seconds, too. So I was high-fiving myself for keeping my goal of progressive improvement, which felt gratifying.

During the first week, my social media was on fire with many in my support team admitting they'd never done core exercises before. It was incredibly encouraging to hear from one female follower who was doing the challenge by starting with just one push-up on her knees, while another male follower shared he was beginning with only three push-ups. People were excited to do this challenge, even those for whom the goal was a bigger physical and mental hurdle than it was for me.

Week 2
The Easier Way to Ab Definition in Two Weeks' Time

By the start of Week 2, I was doing twenty-five push-ups per day and holding my plank for one minute, thirty seconds. It felt awesome to be able to plank for so long, but I admittedly was starting to feel some strain in my lower back when I did so.

Partly because of that, I was now no longer doing the exercises at the same time. The plank, while longer in duration and a bit uncomfortable, was easier for me to do, physically and mentally: it had become habitual to turn on the shower and plank while waiting for the water to warm. But now that the exercise was more tiring, I stopped doing the push-ups immediately after, instead telling myself I'd get to them later in the day.

And for most of the week, I did get to push-ups later in the day, doing them after I got home from the office and had changed out of my work clothes into a T-shirt and scrubs (my equivalent of pajamas). Thank God I had continued my dry month into these first few weeks of February. Even if I did have to go out after work, I didn't drink, which meant I was far more eager to do and capable of doing push-ups when I got home at night.

Yet twice during Week 2, I either forgot to do my push-ups entirely or consciously avoided them. After all, at the end of a fifteen-hour workday, it was exhausting to even consider dropping and giving anyone twenty-five. When I had that internal conversation between myself and my logic about skipping a day, the logic convinced me that by doing so well with my planks I could afford to skip a few push-up reps.

By the end of the second week, I finally saw the first hints of the physical transformation I had experienced with Bar Method. While in the bathroom getting ready for work one morning, I caught a glimpse of myself in the mirror and there it was: my abs looked tighter and more toned, especially my lower abs.

Admittedly, I had been watching my body for any physical change all week, staring at myself whenever I was in front of a mirror like a baker would watch a cake in the oven. But seeing this change was immensely gratifying: despite missing three days of push-ups, all that planking and pushing was finally starting to pay off in more strength and definition.

Week 3
How to Shortchange Back Pain and Get More Core Strength

If Week 3 had a theme, it would have been back pain—and it was definitely all due to the planks. The pain happened only when I was in the position—and went away as soon as I stood up—but it felt pretty unbearable, as if someone had suddenly placed a big weight on the small of my back that radiated pain through my nerves there until I dropped my knees to the floor. I knew I had to change something or give up the challenge, and I couldn't imagine the latter. My support team was counting on me. And I was counting on myself.

But there was an easy solution: modify how I did the planks. There are a number of variations on the standard plank, which is what I had been doing since the start of the challenge—called a forearm plank, you hold your body in a position similar to a push-up, but with both forearms resting on the floor. This is a fantastic way to work your front abdominals, which I'd seen proof of in the mirror the week before, and I wanted to keep doing it, but without holding it for so long that it triggered the torture in my low back.

So I added side planks, sometimes called side bridges, or where you plank laterally, facing one side rather than the floor, with one forearm and the outer edge of one foot on the floor for support. Side planks target your transverse abs and obliques more than the standard plank, so I hoped the variation would not only relieve my low-back pain but also give me a more comprehensive core workout. In other words, I was trading less back pain for rock-star bikini abs, or at least that's what I began to picture during all the planking I was doing. Instead of focusing on the effort, I chose to think of what kind of bikini would look best with my soon-to-be highly toned transverse abs and obliques: Halter top or bandeau? These were important questions to consider while doing planks, obviously.

Midway through Week 3, though, I changed how I planked. Instead of holding a standard plank for as long as possible, I'd plank facing the floor for only thirty to forty seconds, then turn each way to side plank for thirty seconds at a time. This felt so good—all right, "good" may be a bit of an exaggeration, but I had no pain, which was a huge feat—that I repeated the routine once more, planking for a total of three minutes. While I felt a slight ache when holding the standard plank, this lessened if I shifted my weight from side to side on the balls of my feet.

As for push-ups, I was now up to thirty reps total. But as the number increased, so did the physical exertion, and the workout started to feel aerobic rather than simply for strength. In other words, after cranking out thirty consecutive push-ups with good form, I was breaking a slight sweat and breathing hard.

After missing the mark on push-ups twice in Week 2, I was intent to get them out of the way in the morning alongside the planks—no room for procrastination or letting my logic trick me into thinking I was too tired or had already lifted and didn't need more arm exercises. The morning motivation worked six out of the seven days, meaning I missed only one session of push-ups for the week.

At the end of the week, while in the bathroom for my morning mirror scrutiny, I noticed a marked difference in my abs from the week before—more tightness and definition throughout my lower torso. And now, much to my glee, I could see an uptick in muscle tone throughout my arms, with more curve and definition in my biceps, triceps, and deltoids. The only thing I was doing differently were push-ups and planks—nothing new in the gym and no changes to my daily diet.

I was ecstatic. If I was getting such incredible results by doing something that took me less than five minutes per day, why wasn't I making it my mission to keep planking and pushing every day for the entire year? While there were honestly some mornings when push-ups and planks were the last thing I wanted to do, especially the push-ups, I was still doing them—and it was a minor commitment for a major reward.

Over the course of the week, I also realized that I thrived on the sense of accomplishment from this challenge as much as I did on the physical benefits the exercises imparted. I'm sure the endorphin boost I got after thirty push-ups and three minutes planking added something to my elation, but I always felt so fulfilled when I climbed in the shower, knowing I had accomplished something formidable and the day hadn't even started. This, in turn, put me in a good mood all morning, turning this challenge into one where the rewards go beyond physical health.

Week 4
How Just Minutes a Day Can Make You Bikini-Ready in One Month

By the start of the last week, I was up to thirty-seven push-ups and more than three minutes total for my plank routine. I was pleased I was still progressing and hadn't plateaued, but I'd be lying if I didn't admit the push-ups were getting more and more difficult. The numbers were now starting to get a bit intimidating for both exercises, too.

My push-up progression made me feel like a trader watching an IPO on the stock market. How high could I go, baby? I was almost at forty reps, but could I really get up to forty-five by the end of the month? That seemed ridiculously high. Similarly, my plank routine was also starting to feel long—and my bikini dreaming was no longer enough of a distraction. So in addition, I started listening to music, which made the time pass more quickly and kept my brain from focusing on the overwhelming idea of doing forty push-ups or four minutes of planks.

Turns out, the music helped: nothing like a little Bruno Mars to motivate you to hold a front plank for another thirty seconds. But I made a pact with myself now that I would try to add only one more push-up and increase my plank time by only five more seconds before month's end. This was it: I was metaphorically at mile 25 of this month's marathon and I had to finish strong—I didn't want to end up breaking down and walking.

On the very last day of the month, I woke up, had coffee, and turned on the shower per usual . . . and did four minutes, five seconds of planking, followed by forty-six push-ups total. Badass! Physically, I was whipped, but emotionally I was overjoyed. I had just completed an intense five-minute workout I once thought I'd never be able to do, and I was proud of myself for finishing strong, ending the month with a resounding wallop, not a whimper.

My time in front of my mirror that morning came with its own wallop, too. My arms were now back to where they'd been during my Bar Method craze: ripped through my deltoids, triceps, and even chest muscles. My abs looked cut—a word I love to use when complimenting others, but love even more when I can use it about myself—and my posture was much better to boot. I was standing straighter without trying, and instead of pouching out like I loathe, my stomach was holding there flat, muscles fully engaged. I felt stronger and tighter all around, and if *GMA* had wanted to put me in a bikini on national TV, I would gladly have shown off my new body. Okay, maybe not to millions of Americans, but that's how much positive body confidence was now surging through my newly toned physique.

Moreover, I was surprised how easy it had been to get these incredible results in so little time. After all, I had invested only two to five minutes per day in this challenge, and it had transformed my body in a way my normal, hour-long gym routine had never been able to do.

FEBRUARY PUSH-UPS AND PLANKS:
The Science Behind Push-Ups and Planks

M ost strength exercises have plenty of science to prove why you should do them regularly. But push-ups and planks have special merit, research shows, making them a higher priority in your workout routine. Both also require no equipment, fancy gym, personal trainer, class instructor, fitness background, or even significant time commitment.

Push-Ups Work Way More Muscles Than Just Those in Your Chest (Think Abs!)

There's a reason why the push-up has been hailed as "the world's greatest" and most "perfect" exercise by physiologists, athletes, even Harvard University health editors. Push-ups work nearly every muscle in your body, from the tip of your toes to the muscles in your neck, while strengthening tendons, ligaments, and connective tissues, too. The push-up isn't just a good exercise for your arms and chest, as many often assume—the exercise's bigger benefits are recruiting and toning hard-to-strengthen muscles in your back, hips, legs, and abs. Push-ups work large muscle groups, along with smaller, secondary muscles often weak in many people, even trained athletes. Finally, push-ups improve the body's proprioception, or sense of balance, in part by recruiting hard-to-target stabilizer muscles, which help support major muscle groups during movement.

Anyone—Yes, Anyone—Can Do a Push-Up: You Just Have to Know How

Think you can't do a push-up? I'm here to tell you anyone, no matter age, body type, or current strength, can do a push-up. This is an exercise that comes in many shapes and sizes for all our shapes and sizes and doesn't have to be the same excruciating effort you see on TV when some military recruit or fitness buff drops and gives us twenty.

Even if the idea of getting down on your hands and knees is painful, start with a wall push-up, angling your body and keeping your palms firmly flat against the wall while you bend your elbows to bring your chest as close to the wall as possible. You can also try a tabletop push-up: start on your hands and knees with your back flat, then bend your elbows until your nose nearly touches the floor, using your arms and chest to push yourself up. Or try a standard push-up, but with your knees on the floor and your feet slightly suspended above the ground.

If you're a fitness pro, make standard push-ups more challenging by doing them on your knuckles instead of your palms or by using only one arm. You can also add arm-strengthening activities like triceps rows (just grip a dumbbell in each hand) in between reps or try moving your hands closer together so they form a diamond between your index fingers and thumbs. You can do a push-up while balancing on a BOSU ball or keeping your feet on a stability ball. Just remember that, for this month's challenge, the goal is to increase your number of reps, so choose a modification that allows for some progression.

Push-Ups Burn Calories, Trigger Growth Hormones, and Stop Osteoporosis

Cardiovascular exercise isn't the only way to torch calories: studies show strength-training exercises like push-ups are an equally effective way to increase metabolic burn and lose weight. In fact, our bodies burn more calories after strengthening exercises than when we do cardio in order to repair the kind of muscle depletion you get from resistance training. What's more, the more muscle you build from doing exercises like push-ups, the more calories your body burns, at rest or at play.

Resistance exercises like push-ups also stimulate the body's endocrine system to produce more growth hormone, which helps improve physical performance, increases fat loss, and even slows the physical aging process. You'll also boost your body's level of testosterone by doing push-ups—a positive benefit to both women and men, as the hormone is necessary to maintain a healthy metabolism, sex drive, and proper bone mass.

Finally, push-ups are a weight-bearing activity, which means they help stimulate bone growth and repair to prevent osteoporosis. In fact, the AARP even recommends women over age fifty do some form of push-ups daily to help keep healthy bone mass.

Planks Tone More Muscles Than Traditional Ab Exercises

Think of a plank as a pre-push-up. Similarly, planking also provides a full-body workout, engaging a wide range of muscles in your arms, chest, legs, hips, lower back, and abs. In comparison, traditional crunches and sit-ups primarily work only your abs.

But planks also recruit more abdominal muscles than simple sit-ups, crunches, or curls. While these exercises primarily target the rectus abdominis—the muscles that make up what some call the "six-pack"—planks also work your external and internal obliques and stabilizer muscles, along with your transverse abdominis, or the deep muscles that help stabilize the spine and torso. Strengthening all the ab muscles, in turn, helps to better prevent injury, improve performance and posture, and give you better definition throughout your entire stomach.

Planks Isolate Hard-to-Access Core Muscles Better Than Regular Ab Exercises

While the plank is not the only exercise proven by research to strengthen your core, or the muscles in your low back, abs, pelvis, and hips, it is certainly one of the more effective ones. That's partly because the plank is an isometric exercise, meaning you won't change your muscle length or joint angle when you do it. Holding the same position, in turn, forces your body to isolate your core, causing the muscles to work overtime to prevent any movement. And preventing movement, as it turns out, is exactly what the abs were designed to do—support the spine and keep it in one place.

Back Problems? Try Planking Your Way to Pain-Free

Even though I experienced low-back pain while doing the exercise, most experts, including those at the American Council on Exercise, say planking helps prevent back-related aches and injury. That's because the exercise works to strengthen the deep abdominals and muscles surrounding the spine, helping your body better support your back when you exercise, walk, stand, or even sit. Unlike sit-ups, crunches, and most other ab exercises, planking doesn't require your spine to move—in other words, there's no trunk flexion, which can irritate even a minor spinal issue. Planks also don't overdevelop your hip flexors like sit-ups and crunches do, which, in turn, can create pull on the lower back muscles.

Push-Ups and Planks Can Make You Stand Straighter and Look More Elegant

Both push-ups and planks develop muscles that help keep your spine in a neutral position, whether you're resting on the floor or standing up. The stronger these muscles are, the stronger and straighter your spine will be. Push-ups in particular also strengthen the scapula muscles in the upper back, helping keep your shoulders pulled back, not hunched over, while standing or sitting. Finally, strengthening and tightening the deep abdominal muscles helps keep your stomach engaged and flatter when you're walking, standing, or sitting.

Perfect Your Plank

Planking isn't as easy as it looks—it requires good form to get all the benefits described here. Whenever you do a standard plank, your body should form a straight line, from the ends of your heels straight through your legs, butt, back, torso, and head. Don't arch your back or let your hips float toward the floor. If the latter happens, squeeze your glute muscles to prevent your hips from sinking. Keep your palms wide on the floor and don't allow your shoulder blades to cave in, which will add unnecessary strain to your upper body and arms instead of fully engaging your core muscles. Remember to keep your eyes focused on the floor and avoid looking up into a mirror, which can add strain to your neck and low back. Finally, be sure to keep your forearms in line with your shoulders and your feet shoulder-width apart. And don't forget to breathe—holding your breath while planking will only cause the exercise to feel more difficult.

FEBRUARY PUSH-UPS AND PLANKS:
Your Story

You may struggle to find either the time or the motivation to make it to the gym, but I strongly believe everyone and anyone can make two minutes to do push-ups and planks. While this is a no-excuses challenge, there are ways to make it easier and more enjoyable, as I learned. Here are my top ten tips.

1. PUSH AND PLANK FIRST THING IN THE MORNING. Without a doubt, I found it easier to crank out my push-ups and planks first thing in the morning, before leaving the apartment. A morning routine guaranteed I did the exercises instead of waiting and hoping I had extra time during the day or at the gym, didn't have to stay late for work, or wouldn't be too exhausted after I got home. The brain has an interesting way of convincing the body not to do things when we're tired or have already forced ourselves to do too many seemingly unpleasant things, like focus on a work project or give up a run to the vending machine for candy. I personally preferred to do the exercises immediately after I had coffee before I got in the shower, but everyone has a different morning routine. My best advice is to consider push-ups and planks as essential to your morning routine as brushing your teeth. And remember: both activities take just about the same amount of time.

2. PUMP UP TO PUMP OUT. Whether you turn on the radio, use your smartphone, listen to a podcast on your computer, or turn up the volume on your favorite morning TV show, distracting yourself with some music or audible entertainment can help you meet your challenge goals more easily, as I found. Whatever you choose, just be careful not to lift or turn

your head to see a TV, phone, or iPad screen, which can disrupt your form and cause neck and back strain.

3. GET DOWN WITH PPP, A PARTNER FOR YOUR PUSH-UPS AND PLANKS . . . YEAH, YOU KNOW ME! Sharing this month's challenge with a colleague, friend, or family member can keep you on track and motivate you to improve. My PPP was my daughter, Chloe. Granted, she's a Division 1 athlete and she obviously didn't do them with me every single day, but as the month progressed and my reps and duration increased, Chloe helped motivate me to finish strong.

4. REMEMBER THAT YOU'RE DOING SOMETHING THAT TAKES ONLY SECONDS. If your plank duration starts to feel overwhelming like it did with me, think about how many seconds it takes you to hold the position. Because my motto is, if you can still count what you're doing in seconds, it can't be that difficult to do. That's how I approached my push-up number and plank time as the month progressed. Instead of being frazzled by the idea of a four-minute plank, I started to think about it as a 240-second endeavor.

5. FOR EXTRA MOTIVATION, PUSH AND PLANK BEFORE A BIG DATE OR IMPORTANT EVENT. We all know that guy who likes to lift weights right before a big date in hopes of making his arms and chest look bigger. Well, turns out there's some science behind his approach. Doing any kind of exercise that suddenly brings blood into your muscles will make them look more toned. The results don't last long, but I certainly used it as extra motivation those mornings when I didn't want to do the exercises. Since I was usually rushing off to be on *GMA*, I'd tell myself that pushing and planking would make my arms look more defined and my stomach flatter

when I appeared on-air. I confess that not a single viewer wrote in that he or she noticed this, but hey, a girl can dream, right?

6. DON'T BE AFRAID TO MODIFY YOUR PLANK. If you're struggling to hold a standard plank; develop pain or soreness in your back, neck, or shoulders; or simply want to vary your routine, consider adding side planks. Or if you find holding any position too taxing, you can try planking for ten-second intervals, with a short rest in between, which some physiologists say is an even better way to build core strength.

7. START WHERE YOU'RE COMFORTABLE. When I put this challenge out on social media, I received responses from women and men alike who said they were starting with just several push-ups. Others tweeted they could hold a plank for only a few seconds. These responses motivated me because these people were excited to do the challenge and improve, even without the core fitness I already had. It's not about how many push-ups you do or whether your plank time is longer than a friend's. The point of this month—and all the challenges within this book—is to try your best and improve your health and fitness in whatever way you can.

8. RECRUIT A SOCIAL MEDIA SUPPORT TEAM. As was the case with January's dry month, social media helped motivate me to stay strong and finish the month with more push-ups and planks than even I thought possible. Whenever I felt like blowing off the exercises, I'd just check online and see what my friends and followers were sharing and how many reps or how much plank time they'd gained. Knowing we were all enduring the same gritty several seconds together was enough to inspire me to keep going. So share your challenge

with your friends and acquaintances online, and ask them to join you and share their own reps and duration, whether it's just for a day or the entire month.

9. IF YOU CAN FIND A FLOOR, YOU CAN FIND A WAY TO SUCCEED. I've said it before and will do so again: this is a no-excuses challenge. You don't need to go to a gym to do a few push-ups and planks. If there's a floor or ground below you, you have a way to do this challenge.

10. BREATHE. Lots of people hold their breath while exerting themselves—something I learned years ago while training to be an ob-gyn. But holding your breath, whether you're in labor or just trying to do a few push-ups, makes any effort more difficult, increasing pressure in your stomach while decreasing blood flow to your heart, brain, and working muscles. So remember to breathe. Doing so will allow you to add more to your push-ups and planks than you thought possible.

3

Meditation

My Story

About four years ago, I decided I wanted to learn how to meditate. This wasn't a sudden impulse: I'd been hearing from friends, colleagues, and acquaintances for years about how meditating had transformed their lives. But like most Americans, I didn't have a clue how to go about meditating. Should I try sitting cross-legged on the floor and just hope for the best? Was it better to focus on a specific idea or should I try banishing all thoughts from my brain? I had no idea. What I did know was that I was too type A to just wing it, like some of my friends had after a little online research. No, I wanted both an education and an implementable method.

In New York, I connected with Bob Roth, one of the most renowned Americans to teach a type of meditation called transcendental meditation, or TM. The form was first developed by Indian yogis in the 1950s and since has grown to be one of the most widely practiced and well-researched types of meditation in the world. When you practice TM, you sit with your eyes closed for fifteen to twenty minutes twice a day, focusing on a mantra, or calming phrase, you repeat silently. The mantras are supplied to students at different stages of the practice and always kept private.

I signed up for a four-day course in TM at the David Lynch Foundation, where Roth is executive director. During the classes, I learned that I didn't have to control my thoughts while meditating—whatever came into the mind was allowed. This was definitely a *Thank God* moment: given my type A nature, my mind is often a constant film reel of eighty zillion thoughts so the idea of stopping that movie for one minute, let alone twenty, was terrifying.

I also learned that I didn't have to try to control or focus my breath: I simply had a mantra to repeat, and even if that slipped from my mind, that was okay. *I could do this,* I thought. Maybe meditation wasn't that intimidating! After all, tons of people do it, and after four days, I was ready to try myself.

But I still had a few reservations. After the course ended, I asked Roth whether I really had to practice twenty minutes, twice a day. He looked at me and said, "Practice twice a day for two weeks. If you don't feel anything, stop." I must have looked at him inquisitively, because he quickly added, "People don't stop after two weeks, because almost everyone feels so good." That clinched it for me: I was in.

After the course, I meditated every day for nearly a full year. Roth was right: I felt amazing after my two-week trial, with more mental acuity and energy, and less stress, than I had ever experienced. I started with the two twenty-minute sessions daily, but quickly found I could meditate just once every morning and still feel incredible effects.

But all that incredible energy stopped two years ago. Since then

I've allowed my practice to fall by the wayside—and at a time when I needed it the most. Suddenly, I was getting divorced from my husband, who soon thereafter died by suicide, which was an enormous mental, emotional, and even physical blow. In addition, I was experiencing more stress in my professional life, and I just couldn't keep up with the routine. It felt as though I was suffocating, with less and less air coming into my lungs, but I was too breathless to even reach for the oxygen mask I knew was by my side. I missed TM, but at the time, I just couldn't get back into the routine.

In 2017, while speaking at an event in Los Angeles, I ran into Roth, who was also a guest speaker. I shared with him how I'd fallen off my practice and now that things had leveled in my life personally and professionally, I just couldn't seem to find the time to pick it up again, since I was waking up so early to appear on *GMA*. He listened, then asked me what time I thought *GMA*'s coanchor George Stephanopoulos, who practices TM every day, wakes up. I didn't have to think about it—I knew George woke up around 3:30 every morning for the show—a full two hours before my alarm. Could I have gotten up twenty minutes earlier in order to meditate? In his own subtle, effective way, Roth was telling me to stop making excuses. He was right. If George could do it, I could do it.

I vowed to make meditation one of my monthly challenges in 2018. It was the perfect fit, not only for myself but for the thousands of Americans who might join me and had no clue, like I didn't several years ago, about the practice's potentially life-changing effects. Better still, it took only twenty minutes, anyone could do it, and you certainly didn't need to take a course like I did to start practicing.

I decided to make it my mission to meditate for twenty minutes every single day, seven days a week, for an entire month. To be successful, I knew I had to practice this first thing in the morning, before my day started and I got too busy, not waiting until I got home from work, when I knew I'd be too tired. I also preferred morning meditation—it helped immediately establish the right mental energy and mood I wanted for the rest of the day.

Week 1
The Surprising Way Meditation Immediately Changed My Brain

Despite knowing I was about to pick up a practice that would make me feel amazing, I was still slightly anxious on the first day, worried whether I'd really be able to find the time to meditate daily for an entire month. After all, this wasn't like February's challenge where push-ups and planks took me no more than a few minutes in the morning. But I knew my concerns over time were silly—and made me seem like a hypocrite. Whenever patients, friends, or family members say to me they can't find time to exercise or do something beneficial for their physical health, I always respond, *You don't* find *the time, you* make *the time.* I repeated this to myself the first day—and throughout the first week. I was going to *make* the time, because my mental health and mood depended on it.

For the first morning, I set my alarm for 5 A.M. instead of 5:30 A.M. (my normal *GMA* wake-up time), ensuring I'd have plenty of time to meditate and finish my morning routine. Still, when my phone sounded so early in the morning, I felt like chucking the thing and my whole monthly meditation out my New York City apartment window. But I fought the urge and got up anyway, made coffee, and then climbed back into bed, sitting upright on some stacked pillows. The night before, I had downloaded a free meditation app, Insight Timer, which tracks your practice. I hit the start button on my phone, closed my eyes . . . and I did it.

Almost immediately after I opened my eyes, I felt awash in calmness. At the same time, it was as though someone had pumped high-octane fuel into my brain: I felt more focused and mentally energized. I don't suffer from attention deficit disorder (ADD), but the best way I can describe the sensation was that I'd been living with untreated ADD for months and all of a sudden, I was taking the right medication. Shazam! That's how instantly more focused I felt.

For the rest of the day and throughout the first few days, I couldn't believe how much calmer, more focused, and more positive I felt. Daily decisions and difficulties didn't seem to perturb me as much. Traffic on my drive to my medical practice? I could be zen. I also felt like I could go from task to task more efficiently and effectively, with more mental stamina. For example, I didn't have to analyze for hours how I was going to synthesize a complicated health issue for a TV audience or get thrown off by a single letter or bill while charging through a massive pile of mail. If someone had taken a scan of my brain, I'd bet my neurons were now firing faster. And without any medical exam, I knew my levels of cortisol, or the body's stress hormone, were significantly lower, which, in turn, made me less hungry.

That first week, I meditated six of the seven days. I was thrilled and also a bit dumbstruck, now questioning why I had let my practice slip from my life in the first place. I did keep thinking about how I had to wake up thirty minutes earlier for the rest of the month, but I told myself this was only a means to the end. And so far, the end was proving to be mentally marvelous.

Week 2
What Happens When You Meditate Regularly, Then Miss a Day

The second week of my Meditation Challenge, I didn't have to be on *GMA* every single morning. Freedom! Whenever this happens, I feel like I'm back in grade school, getting ready for bed at night knowing the next day is going to be a snow day and celebrating that I don't have to get up so early.

The only problem is that snow days don't tend to make for good meditation days: Without a habitual deadline to get out the door for *GMA*, my mornings lose structure. Instead, I assume I have all the time in the world, which, this week, meant not setting my alarm early to meditate. While this felt like a delicious luxury—sleep, as I realized months later in November's challenge, is one of my most prized commodities—the result was that, by the time it occurred to me that I hadn't done my twenty minutes of zen, I had to bolt out of my apartment to make it into my medical office on time.

At the end of the day, I was disappointed in myself, not only that I'd messed up my challenge but also because I'd spent the whole day feeling less positive and mentally sharp, and noticeably more disorganized. This hadn't happened to me last month when I missed a day of planks and push-ups—there was no noticeable fallout from failing the challenge that day. But not meditating had negative ramifications—and I didn't like it.

That one morning was the only day during the week I didn't meditate—I had learned my lesson. Even though I didn't have a morning routine on weekends, I found it easy to find time to meditate. On Saturdays and Sundays, I had more than sixteen hours, from the time I woke up at 6 A.M. (yes, I'm still an early riser, even on the weekends) until I went to bed around 10 at night, to fit in my practice, with no patients, sometimes no *GMA* segments, and without hundreds of emails to distract me.

I still felt the daily benefits I did the first week: I was more focused, positive, and productive. But now I felt my appetite was increasingly controlled, with fewer cravings and impulsive decisions for unhealthy items. And while it may sound somewhat new age to some readers, after meditating for two weeks, I felt like I'd created this soft cushion between my heart, brain, and body and the harsh stress we all face every day. George Stephanopoulos once described the benefits he gets from meditating this way, and I totally agree.

Week 3
The One Mistake That Will Derail Your Meditation Practice

Even though I now knew skipping my morning practice was a bad idea, I still ended up flagging on two sessions the third week. My first failure was on a weekend—and I had no excuse. I went to bed embarrassed by my slip. It was a shake-my-head kind of moment as I thought to myself, *Are you kidding? What happened?*

The second day I missed was during the workweek—and it was entirely due to an oversight that derailed my practice. I had started to meditate in the morning but didn't set my phone to Do Not Disturb as I always do. And that's like Murphy's Law: whenever you assume someone won't call or text is exactly when they call or text. But instead of ignoring my phone, I opened my eyes and looked over, immediately deciding I had to call back the sender. (I clearly hadn't experienced all the benefits yet from my Mindful Tech Challenge in August.) By the time I got off the phone, I had missed my window to meditate before work.

Similar to the week before, I was angry at myself for missing my practice. Was that phone call really more important than a full day of mental energy and calm? My meditation mistakes were affecting me profoundly, leaving me in a mental and emotional deficit for the day.

Like many people, I live a stressful life, both professionally and personally. On the two days I missed my meditation practice, I was acutely more aware of both kinds of stress in my life. This wasn't because I encountered more difficulties throughout the day—I just couldn't handle the stress that did present itself as well as I did when I meditated in the morning.

The days I did meditate in Week 3, though, I felt more positive, productive, and focused as usual, but also noticeably more able to cope with whatever life threw my way. Annoying emails? No problem. I was also seeing another benefit I didn't feel the first few weeks. Although I'm typically a good sleeper, I can struggle to fall asleep when I'm stressed and also wake up through the night worrying about things. Yet despite what was happening in my life during my Meditation Challenge, the third week in particular, I still slept shockingly well. And the only X factor, or thing I was doing differently, was I was now meditating.

Week 4
How Meditation Helped Me Lose Weight and Gain Empathy

The last week of the challenge, I was determined to meditate every day. I wanted there to be no question whether or not I could do it: I was intent on conquering my meditation month. After all, I had gone four full weeks—and then some—without a single drink during my dry month, so I knew I could do a full week of meditating without one lapse. And I did just that. Yes!

The result: I was amazed how easy it was to practice daily. Better still, you can program your alarm to one time for the full week and never think twice about it. (Okay, maybe I thought twice a few times about getting up at five in the morning, but it was truly worth it). Moreover, I was delighted by how I felt with so much sustained positivity, mental focus, and energy. Without a doubt, Week 4 was one of the best I had had in years, and not because anything wonderful happened or all the stress from the week prior suddenly evaporated. The same difficulties were there, but I was able to handle them more adeptly while feeling happier and upbeat.

Something else happened that week: I started to feel more connected to people. I like to think I'm typically compassionate and connected at my baseline, so it was surprising to feel these emotions amplified. But since I felt more positive and less stressed, I had more patience, understanding, and sympathy for people, even for those I could have a short fuse with in the past.

My sleep continued to be sound, and I had even more mental

energy and focus than the prior week. Interestingly, as my appetite now hovered at basement-floor levels, I felt as though I was starting to lose a little body fat. *What?*, I thought as I started dreaming again about those bikinis I'd imagined during my push-ups and planks month. Is there anything meditation won't help? To think that I'd really been worried about finding the time at the beginning of the month.

While the benefits I felt at the end of the month had been present in earlier weeks, now, after four weeks of consistent practice, they felt accentuated, more highly tuned, and seemed more likely to remain, even if I did miss a morning here or there. I was ending the month physically, mentally, and emotionally healthier, in addition to slightly lighter and leaner.

MARCH MEDITATION:
The Science Behind Meditation

Like many challenges in this book, meditation has a host of health benefits—and too many to enumerate here. Meditation can do so much for your health and wellness, in fact, that many physicians, myself included, prescribe meditation to treat common health conditions, including insomnia, weight gain, and depression. Here are just some of the ways regular meditation can help transform your physical, mental, and emotional health.

Meditation Can Alter Your Genes

Many Americans perceive meditation as a vague activity, with intangible or unquantifiable benefits. They mistakenly presume the only thing that sitting still with eyes closed does is steal time from other potentially more productive activities. Nothing could be further from the truth. And perhaps the strongest evidence of meditation's power is research showing the practice can actually change our genes. According to a number of studies published recently by European researchers, regular meditation suppresses how inflammation is expressed on a genetic level. In other words, meditation practiced over time has the ability to reverse molecular damage on the body caused by inflammation and stress. Some of the genes affected by meditation, according to research, are those commonly treated by overprescribed and potentially harmful anti-inflammatory and pain drugs.

Sleep Problems at Night? Try Meditating in the Morning

I recommend meditation to any and every patient I see with sleep problems, whether they have diagnosable insomnia or just difficulty falling or staying asleep. Those who take my advice tell me that, within weeks of starting to practice, they have fewer sleep difficulties, some patients even more so than when they've used prescription sleep aids in the past. Turns out, meditation is an effective sleeping aid on its own. Studies show regular meditation reduces the number and duration of sleep disturbances, improving overall sleep quality in both people with sleep irregularities and those (like me) who don't typically suffer from sleep issues. What's more, studies show meditation, when practiced regularly, can limit daytime impairment, or feeling tired, slow, and sluggish because you didn't sleep well the night or week before.

Meditation Can Be Just as Effective as Antidepressants

According to 2016 research from Michigan State University and other studies throughout the years, meditation can improve your brain's ability to permanently regulate emotions, making it a just as powerful, if not more effective, antidote for mood problems as many prescription drugs. How does meditation accomplish this? There are several different neuroscientific factors at play, but one reason may be that meditation increases the volume of gray matter in your brain's front cortex while also boosting the size of your right hippocampus. These two areas of the brain are associated with increased emotional control and regulation, along with less stress and more mindful behavior.

Remember how positive I felt on the days I meditated? Turns out, there's scientific evidence for that outcome. Researchers have discovered meditation increases signaling activity in the part of the brain responsible for positive emotions while, at the same time, limiting activity in the side of the brain where negative feelings develop. In simpler terms, the more you meditate, the happier you feel, regardless of life events, simply due to neurocognitive effects. Studies also show meditation boosts self-awareness and feelings of self-acceptance. For all these reasons, regular meditation can treat some depression and anxiety as effectively as prescribed medications, yet without any of the side effects many of these drugs typically carry.

Control Appetite and Lose Weight Effortlessly with Meditation

My goal with the Meditation Challenge never was to lose weight, so I was pleasantly surprised when it happened without any effort, dietary changes, or new workouts. Instead, the practice killed cravings and suppressed my hunger, helping me be lighter and leaner at the end of the month.

Science shows appetite control and weight loss are well-supported benefits of regular meditation. One reason for these effects, researchers who were part of a 2015 study published in the *International Journal of Behavioral Medicine* say, is because meditating better connects you with your body and its physical cues, helping you recognize when you're truly hungry—or when you think you're hungry but the sensation is really a misplaced desire for another mental or emotional need. Meditation also lowers cortisol, a hormone that helps your body store fat and contributes to sugar cravings and overeating. Finally, meditating regularly can boost mood and self-esteem while reducing anxiety and stress, all of which can help you make healthier food choices and prevent or even eliminate emotional or stress-based eating.

Regular Meditation May Make You Smarter

I've never been so focused, productive, and capable of multitasking as on the days when I've meditated. That's in part because meditation increases the brain's gray matter and hippocampus, which not only helps boost mood but also makes your brain bigger, smarter, and more agile. More gray matter and a larger hippocampus also improve your focus, lengthen your attention span, increase your short- and long-term memory, and enhance your ability to multitask and learn new material. A recent study from Yale University also shows regular meditation may alter your brain waves by reducing activity in the neural network that's responsible for mind-wandering thoughts—another reason you may be able to multitask better when you meditate. Other research over the years has also found meditating for just several weeks can improve concentration and attention.

Meditation May Turn Back the Clock on Your Body and Physical Appearance

Numerous studies show that people who meditate regularly have longer telomeres, or caps at the ends of their chromosomes, which are associated with biological age. Every time our cells divide, our telomeres get shorter, so the longer your telomeres, the longer you can likely live, scientists say. What's more, increasing gray matter through meditation may also help preserve your cognitive capabilities well into old age, according to research. Meditating can make you look younger, too, by reducing the stress and inflammation that wreak havoc on skin and hair as well as work internally to physically age us beyond our years.

Help Treat High Blood Pressure, Chronic Pain, and Addiction with More Mindfulness

These conditions are just some of the ailments that science has found meditation can help. In one study, practicing transcendental meditation lowered participants' blood pressure and also reduced their risk of heart attack, stroke, and overall death by any cause. A separate study also found meditation can trigger a big enough blood pressure decrease to allow some participants to safely stop taking hypertension drugs with their doctors' supervision.

As for chronic pain, research shows meditation alters areas in the brain responsible for controlling pain. Some studies suggest practicing regularly can cut chronic pain by as much as 57 percent. Meditation has also shown to be an effective adjunct treatment for drug, alcohol, nicotine, and food addictions and can help alleviate symptoms associated with everything from menopause and the common cold to irritable bowel syndrome and cancer.

Meditation Can Turn You into a Social Butterfly

Meditation is an intensely personal practice that has the ability to make us all more social and better or more deeply connected to those around us, science shows. That's because meditation can help reduce stress and increase feelings of positivity, both of which researchers say can lead to more compassion and empathy for others. Studies have also found meditation can reduce feelings of loneliness. For these reasons, meditation is often prescribed to alleviate and even help treat social anxiety disorder.

MARCH MEDITATION: Your Story

Unlike some challenges, daily meditating requires no physical exertion or dietary discipline. You don't have to drop and do twenty, look the other way at an alluring cinnamon bun, or say no to an appealing glass of pinot. All you have to do is sit quietly for twenty minutes. But I get it: this is still a huge hurdle for many—and it's not necessarily because we're all so busy. Here are ten ways to make meditation part of your day, whether you've never practiced before or have been a yogi all your life.

1. FIND THE RIGHT KIND OF MEDITATION FOR YOU. Transcendental meditation fits my personality, lifestyle, and mood the best, but that doesn't mean it's the right type for you. There are dozens of ways to practice, so talk with friends, do some research, and look online. You may even want to experiment first with a meditation app like Headspace, Buddhify, or Calm, all of which can expose you to different forms of the practice so you can see what works best for you. Some gyms and fitness centers also offer meditation classes, or if you're type A like me, look for courses at your local university or spiritual center. There are also many online courses you can take—just be sure to do a little research first to make sure you go with a reputable site.

2. LEARN HOW TO CHANGE YOUR HEADSPACE. Many Americans have a negative perception of meditation, thinking it simply involves doing nothing for a period of time to attain

some vague, unquantifiable effects. But research unquestionably concludes meditation has a real, profound impact on our physical, mental, and emotional health, even changing how our brains grow and genes function. For this reason, meditation is just as critical to your health and well-being as proper hygiene, exercise, and diet. Would you go a day without brushing your teeth? Meditation should be as nonnegotiable as this.

3. CONSIDER MEDITATION AN INVESTMENT IN YOUR DAILY PRODUCTIVITY. I can't reiterate how much more focused and productive I felt during the days I meditated in the morning. If you think you don't have time to meditate, I guarantee if you take just twenty minutes to try it, you'll discover you'll make the time up tenfold by being more productive, focused, and effective the rest of the day. The majority of the busiest and most successful people I know in the world meditate daily, if not twice daily. Learn from their example.

4. SET YOUR ALARM THIRTY MINUTES EARLIER. This is the easiest and most effective way for many to make meditation a daily habit—it's certainly the best method for me and others I know who meditate regularly. Otherwise, it's all too easy to get busy and preoccupied with professional and personal obligations, as you put meditation on your mental back burner until you realize it's too late and the day is over. Once you get out and start your day, it can also be difficult to slow down, mentally and physically, in order to get into the proper headspace to sit still for twenty minutes. Finally, there's a huge benefit to morning meditation: it boosts positivity, productivity, and overall mood, setting you up to embrace the day as soon as you open your eyes from your practice.

5. DEDICATE A REGULAR SPACE TO MEDITATE. This can be critical to your monthly success if you live with a spouse, children,

roommates, or needy pets. Before the month begins, choose a place in your home where you won't be disturbed and where you can meditate every morning. Knowing you have a go-to spot on the first day will also make the practice less intimidating and easier to adopt. I mostly meditated in my bed, where I was never disturbed by my kids or dog, Mason. Also, like any other habit, establishing consistency is the best way to turn a new practice into a daily custom.

6.   DON'T BE AFRAID TO MEDITATE OUTSIDE THE BOX—OR OFF THE BED. While I strongly believe morning meditation is the best way to make the practice a daily habit, there are inevitably those days when you can't wake up thirty minutes early or meditate before you leave the house, like in the instance of a superearly flight. But as I've discovered, if there's a will, there's a way. For example, in the instance of an early flight, I've found meditating on airplanes is easy and immeasurably beneficial, helping to alleviate both the boredom and the stress of air travel.

If you have to rush out the door for an early meeting, there's nothing wrong with meditating in the office. When I do it, I shut the door and put a Do Not Disturb sign on it to let people know I'm busy, and I silence the ringer on my office phone and mobile, as well as email alerts on my computers.

Another good spot for a spontaneous meditation session is in the car. I've meditated there many times while waiting to pick Chloe up from a hockey game. You can also meditate in a quiet room or a closed-door yoga studio at your gym or fitness center, which some people find convenient to do after a workout. Finally, meditating outside on a beach, in a park, or even in your own backyard can be peaceful and conducive to your practice. Remember, what's more important than where you do it is doing it in the first place.

7. PUT YOUR PHONE ON DO NOT DISTURB. Don't gamble with
    your time like I did once during my challenge by forgetting
    to turn off your phone. You may assume no one will call, text,
    or email you in the morning, but it's a risk you don't need
    to take, especially if you go through the effort of waking up
    early. Moreover, getting interrupted by a beep, ding, or ring
    when you're meditating is particularly jarring—and no way
    to start your day. Nearly any call or text can wait twenty min-
    utes until you finish your practice.

8. USE A MEDITATION TIMER. No matter which type of med-
    itation you choose, use a timer so that your practice has
    structure. A timer, whether you download an app to your
    phone, use a stopwatch, or set a traditional kitchen timer,
    will allow you to focus fully on your practice, preventing
    your mind from wondering how long you've been sitting or
    how much longer before you can open your eyes.

9. SHARE YOUR PRACTICE WITH OTHERS. Telling the people you
    love and trust in your life that you're meditating can help
    you feel proud of your practice and reinforce the positivity
    that meditation brings. During my Meditation Challenge,
    my only regret was not telling more friends, colleagues, and
    patients that I had started to practice again. If I had, it not
    only would have added even more energy to the challenge,
    it also would have corroborated my commitment to doing it
    daily. And as I learned during my dry month and through-
    out the year, announcing any challenge out loud to friends
    and family makes the mission more real while increasing
    your accountability to see it through.

10. PRACTICE COMPASSION WITH YOURSELF. Meditation is not
    necessarily easy for everyone. For some, it's a foreign con-
    cept that causes anxiety as you struggle with what to do and

how to do it. But I strongly believe that anyone can meditate, and as long as you're attempting to calm your mind, then you're accomplishing your goal, no matter what any yogi or instructor says. Don't beat yourself up if you get restless. Leverage the compassion meditation teaches and turn it inward. If anything, use your practice to learn how to be kind to yourself and grant yourself permission to fail. Meditating, at its very base, is about creating self-love, not new reasons to feel like a failure. Even if you simply have the desire to meditate, you're already halfway there, accomplishing the practice's intent of opening your heart to yourself and new possibilities.

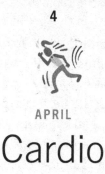

4

APRIL

Cardio

My Story

Exercise is oftentimes the most difficult challenge for anyone who wants to improve their health and look and feel their best. I get it: working out on a regular basis is not easy. It takes physical, mental, and emotional self-discipline, along with commitment, schedule structure, and a consistent attitude to get it done. I've been fortunate enough to possess those traits and have worked out regularly for most of my life. And perhaps most important, I actually like exercise. But two years ago, I decided to stop doing nearly all cardiovascular exercise, which surprised me, as both a fitness enthusiast and a physician who prescribes aerobic exercise to all my patients.

It didn't happen because I woke up one morning and suddenly decided that all the cycling, running, swimming, and cardio classes I was doing weren't important to my overall health anymore. Or that I was bored with these aerobic workouts and couldn't find the motivation. On the contrary, I was still going to the gym at least five days per week—a daunting and herculean feat for most people.

The reason I stopped doing cardio was simply for vanity. Here I was, working out almost every day for at least an hour at a time, doing what I thought was the perfect combination of cardio, with some resistance training and high- and low-intensity days, and I still didn't have the strong, defined look I wanted.

One day, as I walked into a fitness class, I grabbed the instructor, Cliff Randall, who later became my personal trainer, to ask his advice. When I detailed what I'd been doing, he didn't hesitate: he thought I was doing *too much* cardio exercise. I was surprised, but as he explained it, high-intensity aerobic exercise burns the body's readily available glycogen—or the carbohydrate stored in your muscles and liver—rather than your fat stores. To lean down, he said, I needed to do workouts like heavy weight training that would quickly deplete my glycogen stores so my body could tap into its fat supply. If I were going to do cardio, which is key for heart and brain health, he suggested a longer-duration, lower-intensity session. On his advice, I stopped doing endurance workouts and started lifting heavy weights, only jumping on the treadmill or a spin bike to warm up my body before lifting.

After a year of following Cliff's suggested routine, I had more lean muscle mass, but sorely missed all the physical and mental benefits that cardio exercise had once afforded me. I knew I had lost fitness—a good set of stairs, usually taken in four-inch heels, now socked my lungs and heart more than it should—and I wasn't processing stress as well as when I was taking out my angst on a good, sweaty bike ride or run. I also wasn't able to lift as often as I could bike, run, or take cardio classes—lifting with heavy weights taxes your muscles more than aerobic exercise—and I felt like, while I had more lean muscle now, my workouts were beginning to slide, with twelve months of hard lifting taking its toll on my muscles, tendons, and ligaments. And at a certain point, you can only have so much muscle mass, so continuing to lift heavy weights nearly every day can have diminishing returns.

I also missed sweating. I know that may sound odd to some, but for my entire life, I've always done some form of cardiovascular exercise. In high school, I played field hockey and lacrosse, with lots of running and other endurance training to stay competitive. When I was in medical school, aerobic exercise was the most effective way for me to relieve stress—and I know it prevented me from catching all the colds and other illnesses most students and residents came down with from spending too much time in hospitals and getting too little sleep.

But working aerobic exercise back into my weekly routine after a year hiatus seemed formidable. When I had tried before beginning my Cardio Challenge, vowing to go to a spin class or run on the treadmill after work, I often failed, opting for weights instead, which seemed to require less effort after a long day. I started to grow concerned: Would I ever get back to cardio?

For these reasons, I decided to make aerobic exercise one of my monthly challenges, which I knew would reverberate with just about everyone in my life. So many of my patients, friends, and colleagues, along with followers who were vocal about their dread of aerobic exercise, don't work out enough, if at all. While exercise has been part of my lifestyle for years, I realize that, for most people, working out is extremely difficult! Getting to the gym or going for a run feels like an immense challenge, and for some, it also means physical pain, body shame, mental boredom, or just plain anxiety. Then there's the time factor: with all the other obligations we have in life, I understand that many people struggle to simply find the time to work out.

So while my motivation for this month may have been distinctly personal—to get back to doing what I love and know I need for my overall health—I knew the challenge of simply trying to do any type of aerobic exercise would benefit so many people. To that end, I decided I wanted to structure the challenge so that anyone, no matter their current fitness level or lifestyle, could join. I made it my goal—and suggested to anyone who wanted to join me—that the mere point of the month would be to do some type of cardio activity that elevated your heart rate for twenty minutes most days of the week. This didn't have to be a heart-pounding run or a sweaty session in the gym; it could be a brisk walk around the block, dancing to your favorite music in your living room, or taking the time to replant your spring garden beds.

I was excited to kick off the month, but also anxious: I hadn't done any aerobic exercise other than a ten-minute warm-up on a bike or treadmill in more than a year. I was also concerned that I would miss lifting weights, since I knew I wouldn't have time to fit in a longer aerobic workout alongside weights most days of the week. I figured I could do more push-ups and planks, though, now that I knew how well they worked to keep me toned in such little time.

When I announced the challenge on social media, the response was slightly more reluctant than what I'd received to the year's previous challenges. While many responded that they knew they should get in aerobic exercise, I also heard how difficult it was to do or find time for. Clearly, this was a challenge everyone, me included, needed badly.

Week 1
How Sweating More Helped Me Stress Less

On Day 1, I went charging out of the gate, signing up for a forty-five-minute SoulCycle class with one of my favorite instructors, Julie Dermer. I'd taken the spin classes regularly before and loved them. You don't have to think but can just show up while the instructors lead you through different rpms, movements, and music—afterward, you leave sweaty and full of endorphins. The only hiccup is, in New York City, you have to sign up and pay for the class beforehand, which means once you commit, there's no backing out unless you want to lose $36.

The first day, I purposely went early so I could get a bike in the back of the studio. Usually, I like to ride in the front because it motivates me to ride harder and get more out of the class with seventy-some pairs of eyeballs on my back. But today, I didn't want anyone watching me in case I couldn't keep up.

As it turns out, my fear of failure was baseless—I loved every minute of the class. I wasn't as fit as I was a year ago and nor could I ride as hard as I could a year ago, but I loved being back on the bike, singing along with the music, and cycling with the rhythm of my own spinning. When I got off, I was dripping with sweat and surging with endorphins—two things you don't get after lifting weights. Walking out of the studio afterward, I thought to myself that if this was how the month was going to proceed, I'd be just fine.

I wanted to vary my workouts so I wouldn't burn out, physically or mentally, so the next day I decided to swim. This was a bigger commitment for me than taking a spin class. In my mind, swimming requires a greater level of fitness—and the ability to propel yourself through water without being able to breathe freely. The workout is also psychologically challenging, requiring a lengthy preprocess of changing and showering before you can even start. Then there was my personal hang-up: I really don't like the feeling of walking on wet pool decks. It grosses me out.

But several years ago, while training for a triathlon, I grew to really enjoy swimming. It was a different type of workout, with a different type of aftereffect, than any exercise I'd done. When you get out of the pool after a good lap session, you can feel every part of your body, inside and out, pulsing with activity. There's no other activity like it that I've ever tried.

In New York, I belong to a gym near my apartment that has a small three-lane pool. Despite being a member there for years, I'd never once used the pool, but on Day 2, I headed to the gym, suited up, padded across the dreaded wet cement, and spent fifty minutes swimming laps. This I broke up into ten-minute training blocks, with ten minutes each of swimming freestyle, with flippers, with hand paddles, with a pull-buoy, et cetera, to break up the monotony and target different muscle groups.

I was elated when I got out of the pool. As much as I disliked the process and prep of swimming, I had forgotten how much I enjoyed being underwater. And the workout didn't feel anything like the SoulCycle class I took the day before. For one thing, it wasn't a dark room, with club-quality music and a disco ball. Instead, my lungs were taxed in a way they hadn't been in years, and I could feel every fiber in my muscles when I finished. It was almost as if I wasn't even doing the same type of exercise—aerobic—as the day before, which was something I never felt when I switched up my routine while lifting.

I'd enjoyed the swim session so much that I opted for laps again for my next workout, with another fifty minutes in the pool. Next was a fifty-five-minute, then forty-minute ride on the stationary bike in the small gym in my apartment building complex. I don't love the facility, but when I'm pressed for time, I can't beat the convenience of taking an elevator down to the basement for a quick workout. The stationary bike was satisfactory, but it's difficult to push myself as hard as I do in SoulCycle class. I also got bored on the bike without the variety of including movements or the energy of an instructor like Julie to motivate me along.

When the week ended, I had done only five aerobic workouts, not the six I had hoped for. But I wasn't disappointed at all. I had gone longer all five days than the twenty-minute minimum I'd set, and I liked that I'd managed two days in the pool, too. I also lifted weights for an hour one day when I didn't do cardio and tried to fit in some morning push-ups and planks, so I was pleased I'd still found time for resistance training.

More important, I felt more physically and psychologically relaxed than I had in a long time before last month's Meditation Challenge. Five endurance workouts were already starting to sap stress, and combining meditation in the morning with a daily aerobic workout was like a double whammy of amazing for my mood. I also surprisingly felt more toned throughout my entire body, not just strong in the muscles I lifted during a strength workout. And while I'm generally a good sleeper, midway through the week, after just three cardio workouts, I started to sleep more deeply and soundly.

Week 2
Finding New Ways to Work Out While Traveling

I started the second week with an uninspiring hour on the stationary bike in my apartment gym. While this was my longest cardio session to date since starting the month, I was spinning at such a low intensity that it didn't feel challenging. Instead, I was bored—I felt like I was riding only to move my legs—but I was still pleased I'd fit the workout in.

The next day, it was back on the bike, this time for forty-five minutes, while I opted to go to the gym later in the day to lift weights. It had been a rare day because I didn't have to see patients at my medical office, and it felt like an extraordinary luxury to be able to do two workouts in one day. So while the bike hadn't been a memorable workout, the overall day was exhilarating since I had the chance to get a little endorphin rush, along with that great tough-girl boost I get after lifting weights.

For the rest of the week, I was in Los Angeles on a work trip. The day I flew out, I purposely decided to take off from any exercise. I strongly believe we all need one day off per week, and mine are more reactive than intentionally planned—that is, I realize I'm too busy at work or with travel to find time for a twenty-minute trip to the gym.

The good thing about going to L.A., though, was that I'd stayed many times at the same hotel and knew there was a SoulCycle studio only steps away. A whole new set of instructors and teaching styles from what I was accustomed to in New York was exciting, too, and I booked a class for the day after I landed with my favorite L.A.-based SoulCycle instructor, Edward Pagac.

Turns out, the L.A. studio was everything I had remembered it to be since I'd taken my last class there months ago. After my unremarkable rides in my apartment gym, being in a new studio was thrilling, as was the class itself, and I was pumped to leave sweating and full of endorphins. I decided to go to classes the next two consecutive days before I flew back to New York.

The day after I landed back home, I wrapped up the week with a fifty-minute swim—a critical component of variety after a week straight of cycling and spinning. I had logged six cardio workouts total, along with one day in the weight room. This felt amazing: despite a crazy travel schedule, I had still managed a productive and diverse week, with three high-intensity spin classes, two low-intensity stationary bike rides, and a swim to boot.

At the end of the week, I noticed that I had more energy than I had had in weeks. My stress levels continued to be lower than they had been in the months before my Meditation Challenge. Interestingly, I also felt slimmer now, as though as I was tighter throughout my body and lighter on my feet. With a break from heavy lifting, I also felt more limber and efficient. Why had I ever stopped doing cardio again?

Week 3
How to Catch the Cardio Bug and Turn Exercise into a Daily Habit

After a demanding week of work, travel, and seven gym sessions total, I was beat and needed a rest, physically and mentally. I felt like I deserved some downtime and a glass of wine (and I did have

one glass, not an oversize pour, thanks to my January Dry Challenge), not a prolonged trip to the gym. So I started the third week
with another intentional day off, booking a SoulCycle class for the
following day, guaranteeing I'd get right back into it.

I was enjoying SoulCycle and most of my time on the stationary bike, but I knew I had been avoiding one workout I wanted to
include this month: running. Like many people, I have a love-hate
relationship with running. I used to jog often when I was training for a triathlon—and loved it—but I stopped after I developed
Achilles tendonitis. Since then my Achilles can flare up when I
run, although I've learned to mitigate injury by jogging for only
short distances and sticking to the treadmill, which is more for-
giving than tarmac or cement. I'm also not as comfortable running as I am cycling or spinning—it's physically demanding in a
way that my body isn't built for.

But I wanted to try it and did so this week, logging my first run
in years by doing thirty-five minutes on the treadmill, alternating
between one minute of jogging and one minute of brisk walking.
Afterward, I felt great, breathing harder than I had in SoulCycle
and enjoying a similar, if not even bigger, endorphin high. Better
still, I didn't feel my Achilles at all.

After this big aerobic boost, I spent the next day cycling for forty-
five minutes in my building at such a low intensity that I returned
emails and texts from the bike. I didn't usually like to do this—
when I'm working out, I want to unplug and work my body, not do
my work—but I felt a multitasking ride was better than nothing
at all, which would have been the case if I couldn't use the time to
catch up with patients.

To make up for my slack workout, I lifted the next day for an
hour, followed by a forty-minute run-walk on the treadmill. Although I felt more energetic and slimmer from my aerobic exercise
than I had in a year, I missed weight lifting and that tough feeling
I got after pushing around some heavy weights.

The following day, I wanted to go to SoulCycle, but there were no classes that fit my schedule. Admittedly, I'm also picky and usually will only take classes taught by my two favorite New York–based instructors, James Jarrott and Julie; if I can't get to one of their classes, I usually don't go. But since I wasn't excited to return to my apartment-building bike, I decided to ride one of the spin bikes at my regular gym that they keep in a studio separate from the rest of the facility. Once there, I was the only one in the room, which turned out to be marvelous for a workout. All alone and surrounded by mirrors, I felt like an elite athlete in my own private studio, watching myself stay determined to break a sweat and get in a high-high-intensity workout. I rode for an hour, first listening to music, then to a podcast, which I had never done before while working out.

I rounded out the week with a third session on the treadmill, this time for thirty minutes. I had caught the running bug again and didn't want to stop. I would have jogged longer had I not been concerned about irritating my Achilles ahead of a weekend when I'd spend lots of time on my feet at Chloe's hockey games.

At the end of the week, I was surprisingly pleased by how much aerobic exercise I'd been able to fit in so far for the month. I couldn't believe I was swimming, running, and biking—and even lifting some weights. I admittedly missed not being able to find more time to strength train, and I knew my challenge going forward would be to find a way to fit both aerobic and resistance training into my daily routine.

Week 4

Cracking the Code for a Better Body (Hint: It's Not About Weight Loss)

I kicked off the last week with what I call a check-the-box workout, doing thirty minutes in my apartment gym just to get in an aerobic workout. The day had been hectic, and I didn't particularly enjoy the ride physically or mentally, but it was a workout, still burning calories and imparting benefits I wouldn't get if I had opted just to sit at my laptop or waste time on social media.

Knowing I needed a more inspiring workout, I headed back to the spin studio at my gym the following day. This time, I listened to a podcast for the entire hour-long ride. This was new territory: While I had always enjoyed music while working out, I never once thought hearing spoken words would inspire me. Yet here I was, listening to an episode from *Wine Enthusiast* of all things, and loving it. I was so excited to be learning something while working out—multitasking at its best—that I didn't even realize I had ridden for an hour until I looked down at my watch.

The next two days, I returned to SoulCycle to get a double hit of intense aerobic workouts. After I left the second class all sweaty and sore, I was proud of myself for alternating between hard and easy days, with the high intensity of SoulCycle to boost my fitness and get lean, and the low intensity of easy spin days that would help maintain fitness and burn calories.

The last weekend of the month, I went away on a spring ski weekend and tried snowshoeing for the very first time. I couldn't believe how much I enjoyed it. I thought I'd spend most of the time falling over in the snow, but the movement was more instinctual than I'd imagined while the workout itself was far more challenging. I spent the entire hour breathing hard and sweating despite the cold, trying to move my feet as quickly as possible so I didn't sink in the snow. Meanwhile, I was motivated by everything I saw as the beauty of being outside in the deep quiet of the winter woods sunk in.

To end my challenge, I spent the next day downhill skiing. I couldn't think of a better way to wrap up my cardio month. I hadn't been skiing in years—and I've missed some great slope-style fashion as a result. While my outfit might have been out of date, after four weeks of consistent endurance training, I was in better shape and condition to spend hours at a time out on the mountain.

Initially, I had been worried about what all this cardio would do to my physique. But at the end of the month, I had actually lost a pound or two. This was despite the fact that I had eaten more fig and prosciutto pizza—my favorite indulgence when I let myself eat carbs—than I had in years.

My energy levels also felt at least 15 percent higher than normal. Thanks, SoulCycle! I continued to have an easier time sleeping and felt more mentally sharp as a result. More so, I felt healthier than I had in the months when I was just lifting weights—my brain, lungs, heart, skin, and every other organ had benefited immensely from this challenge. But most of all, the month had taught me something I already knew but had lost sight of: we need aerobic exercise *and* weight training to stay healthy, fit, and lean. One or the other isn't the secret to the perfect body, but like everything else in life, a balanced, moderate approach to both will give you the physical, mental, and aesthetic benefits you want. Because at the end of the day, no matter your shape or size, a fit, healthy body is a perfect body.

APRIL CARDIO:
The Science Behind Cardio

You likely know aerobic exercise is imperative to health. Our bodies were designed to move, and we need physical activity to function optimally—without running after our prey or at least walking to the store, we're at a much greater risk of developing chronic diseases like cancer, heart disease, stroke, arthritis, and other ailments. Exercising may be a tough habit to pick up, but not incorporating some type of aerobic exercise on a regular basis can also lead to weight gain, obesity, and skin and hair problems. Here are other surprising benefits of simply raising your heart rate and sweating more.

Avoiding Aerobic Exercise May Be as Bad for Your Health as Smoking

Lots of my health-minded friends, patients, and colleagues are horrified by the idea of smoking cigarettes. But many don't do any or enough cardio activity, which studies show can be just as detrimental to your overall health as smoking. In fact, a 2012 study published in *The Lancet* even found that physical inactivity can lead to as many deaths worldwide as smoking. That's because aerobic exercise, whether a regular gym routine, walking your dog, or doing strenuous housework, has been shown to lower the risk of nearly every chronic disease. For this reason, research shows people who exercise live longer than those who don't. Moreover, those who are physically active live better later on in life—with less chronic pain and more day-to-day enjoyment—than those who don't exercise regularly.

Raise Your Heart Rate to Get Smarter Overnight

Cardio has some amazing benefits for your brain. Not only does it help decrease the risk of cognitive diseases like Alzheimer's, Parkinson's, and early-onset dementia, aerobic exercise also helps boost the size of your brain's hippocampus, responsible for learning and memory. People who regularly do cardiovascular activity, studies show, have better memory skills than those who stick to strength training or do no exercise at all. Aerobic exercise also works to reduce insulin and systematic inflammation, both of which can have a negative effect on cognitive performance, while triggering the growth of new brain cells. This, in turn, is one reason why researchers have found that a good sweat session can help increase your focus for up to three hours, while also improving your brain's ability to prioritize and conceive of new ideas.

Worried About Breast Cancer? Slash Your Risk with Sweat Sessions

Many of my patients are worried about breast cancer—and rightfully so. But one of the best ways to prevent the disease is by doing regular exercise, which studies show can help reduce your risk by up to 40 percent. In fact, a study published in 2017 in *Canadian Medical Association Journal* found that doing more aerobic exercise is the best way women with breast cancer can prevent reoccurrence, even more effective than making dietary changes. Credit cardio's amazing effects to the fact that it reduces estrogen levels, along with the amount of estrogen-sensitive tissue in a woman's breasts. Exercise also lowers insulin and shrinks fat cells, reducing the likelihood of cancer growth.

Use the Gym to Treat High Blood Pressure and Cholesterol

One in three Americans has high blood pressure, while one in three also has high cholesterol. This has produced a country of medicated men and women, which is often necessary and appropriate since these drugs save lives. But both blood pressure and high cholesterol are largely treatable with lifestyle modifications like aerobic exercise and a healthy diet, and these adaptations should always come before resorting to prescription medications.

While some causes of high cholesterol and hypertension are genetic or stem from internal factors not related to what we do or eat, a large majority of high blood pressure and cholesterol cases can be prevented by exercise. In fact, according to the Mayo Clinic, being active can reduce systolic blood pressure as much as some medication. Similarly, a study of ten thousand people that appeared in *The Lancet* in 2012 found the fittest people who didn't take statins were 50 percent less likely to die from a heart event than those taking statins but who didn't exercise. The problem is that most people would rather take a drug than get to the gym.

A recent University of North Carolina at Chapel Hill study found that just 12 percent of Americans have optimal numbers for blood pressure and cholesterol, along with other heart disease indicators like blood sugar, triglyceride levels, and waist circumference. In other words, we are doing very poorly on our "metabolic" report cards, and the treatment for everyone, even if you don't have clinical high blood pressure or cholesterol, is more exercise.

Why You Can't Be Lean *and* Healthy Without Aerobic Exercise

Despite the misinformation I once received, aerobic exercise is an effective way to lose weight and get lean. While my trainer was absolutely right that resistance training adds muscle tone and definition, and too much cardio can thwart weight-loss efforts, aerobic exercise helps anyone lose weight more quickly and better keep that weight off over time. Not only does cardio exercise blast calories and rev metabolism, it also improves your body's ability to tap into and burn fat, even physically shrinking fat cells over time. As I learned, the best way to lose weight and get or stay lean is to combine both cardio and resistance training.

Sweat Just a Little to Look Younger Instantly

Aerobic exercise won't just make you lean and more energetic, it can also shave years off how you look and feel—and not just because it helps prevent disease. Studies show that cardio may actually reverse the aging process on a cellular level, triggering changes in skin cells that help you look younger than your physical age.

A 2014 study from McMaster University even found people who started exercising after age forty had skin characteristics on a cellular and epidermal level more similar to twenty- and thirty-year-olds than individuals their own age. Endurance exercise also increases the flow of blood, oxygen, and nutrients to skin, which helps improve its overall health, elasticity, and appearance.

Aerobic Exercise May Be the Best Sleeping Pill You Can Swallow

I have lots of patients who suffer from sleeping problems, and the majority of the time, their difficulties could be improved simply by being more active throughout the day. Doing as little as ten minutes of aerobic exercise on a regular basis drastically improves a person's ability to fall asleep and stay there, according to the National Sleep Foundation. Not only does cardio exercise in particular increase sleep quality and duration, it also reduces stress and fatigues the body, physically and mentally. Multiple studies even show aerobic exercise is effective at treating clinical insomnia. If you suffer from sleeping problems, try to exercise in the morning or afternoon, since studies show aerobic activity right before bed can cause wakefulness.

APRIL CARDIO: Your Story

For many readers, this month's challenge will be the most difficult one to complete in the entire year. While physical exertion isn't necessarily easy, the dread of working out is almost always far worse than the actual workout. The uplifting feeling you get after you finish a bike ride, brisk walk, jog, or cardio class is inimitable—one reason why no one ever regrets working out. And the more you exercise over time, the easier and more enjoyable it gets. You might even find yourself addicted to aerobic activity like I am. Here are ten ways to nail this month's challenge and turn aerobic exercise from a chore into an everyday addiction.

1. START BY TELLING YOURSELF THAT ANYTHING IS BETTER THAN NOTHING. If you're new to exercise, enthusiasm is a great thing, but if you begin the month by running an hour every day, six days a week, you'll likely burn out quickly or get injured. Remember, any aerobic activity is better than nothing, so even twenty minutes of brisk walking can fit the bill when you don't feel like going out the door. For those days when you're really not motivated, tell yourself to do only five minutes of exercise. Chances are, once you're out the door or at the gym and moving, you'll likely feel more energized and want to keep going longer than you expected.

2. FIND SOMETHING YOU LOVE. Not all cardio is created equal. If you don't like aerobic exercise, it might be that you just haven't found the right workout for you. I like to swim, jog, bike, and take cardio classes like SoulCycle. (My bank account, however, may *not* like it, but I tell myself the investment in my health is worth it.) However, I have friends who love working out but wouldn't set foot in a gym because they'd rather be outside, hiking, biking, gardening, or walking. Others like to dance, box, play on a local adult sports team, jump rope, or do exercise videos at home or even climb stadium stairs while waiting for their kids at school. If there's a type of aerobic exercise you already enjoy, that's fantastic. But if not, experiment by trying different gyms, classes, and outdoor and indoor sports. And don't be afraid to think outside the box to less traditional cardio activities like ballroom dancing, squash, Rollerblading, or water aerobics.

3. PLAN AHEAD. Any new lifestyle adaptation takes planning. At the beginning of the month, I printed out a paper copy of my

weekly calendar and studied it like a map to figure out when I could fit in a workout each day, considering whether I would have time to get to and from a SoulCycle class or whether it'd be safer to opt for the gym in my apartment building. Planning my workout in advance also meant I could pack a gym bag before work or bring along my swimsuit for the pool.

An easier option, if you don't have an early-morning commitment like I do, is to exercise in the morning. This way, no matter what happens to your day—if you have to stay late at the office, get suckered into a postwork happy hour, or simply feel exhausted after a long day—you've already done your aerobic exercise. Research shows people who work out first thing in the morning exercise more regularly and continue the habit for a longer time than those who work out at other times in the day.

4. MIX IT UP. I would have struggled with this challenge if I only ran or swam or biked. Having different aerobic options prevents physical and mental burnout. The same goes for workout duration and intensity. Don't expect to do a ninety-minute boot camp class or high-intensity run every day—and you shouldn't try, as the body needs more than twenty-four hours to recover from long, endurance, or intense workouts. At the same time, avoid doing only low-intensity workouts, which can prevent physical fitness gains and stall weight loss.

5. CREATE ACCOUNTABILITY. One reason I did a lot of SoulCycle for my cardio challenge month is that the classes held me more accountable to my mission. Once I signed up, I was unlikely to skip the class because I had already paid $36, which is an expensive way to spend forty-five minutes. And once in class, I wasn't going to quit early and walk out in front of the instructor and other participants. Group-exercise classes aren't the only way to create accountability, either. Arrange

to meet a friend for a morning run or plan a lunch-hour bike ride with a colleague. Or if you're the type motivated by the idea of not wasting money, join a new gym or pay for a bundle of classes at a boutique exercise studio.

6. TAP INTO YOUR SOCIAL MEDIA TEAM. While I didn't need motivation to work out per se—I was already exercising most days of the week—I did need help doing aerobic exercise again. That's why I told my friends and followers on social media that I was doing a cardio challenge. This not only made me more accountable but also produced some inspired tweets and comments that I read whenever I thought my bed looked better than a bike. I highly recommend you also share your challenge goals and the details of your daily workouts with your social media team. Friends may decide to join you or share their own workout stats, which can help inspire you to get to the gym. Social media can also help you discover new workout routines, exercise options, and motivational tips.

7. TRACK IT. Keeping a record of what type and how much cardio you do can inspire you by providing a visual account of your success to date. I wrote down how long and which kind of workout I did on a paper calendar for the entire month, so I could hold it in my hands and see what I was accomplishing. Some days I think I even worked out solely so I could log another day. If you're more motivated by tech, there are tons of apps that allow you to track your workouts or compare your routine with friends or another group, which can make you feel part of a team.

8. TARGET A SPECIFIC GOAL LIKE A RACE OR A NEW SPORTING SKILL. Some people are more motivated to exercise when they have a specific event to train for, like a 5K race or a

mini-triathlon, or they decide to try to accomplish a new skill or feat, like learning to surf or losing ten pounds. To pair your cardio challenge with a particular goal, consider what matters to you, whether you want to play a new sport, compete in an event for yourself or for a philanthropic cause, check off a bucket-list item like running a marathon, or slim down for a special occasion like a vacation or a reunion. Enlist a trainer or look online for training plans or other resources to help you meet your goal. If you're trying to lose weight, combine your cardio with some diet modifications like cutting out processed foods and reducing sugar for more effective and sustainable results.

9. MOVE BEYOND MUSIC. I loved working out to music and didn't think there was any reason to try anything else—until my Cardio Challenge, when I started listening to podcasts during spin sessions. Unlike music, podcasts or audiobooks provide a narrative or conversation that you can focus on while working out, passing the time and providing a distraction from the physical effort. When I listened to an educational podcast, whether it was on wine or something more serious like politics or history, I loved the idea that I was improving my mind while bettering my body.

10. DO IT FOR YOUR INSTAGRAM ACCOUNT. Taking a scenic bike ride, trying something new like a dance class or flag football, going for a trail run, hiking, or even harvesting your garden bounty are excellent photo opportunities—and sharing pics of your cardio journey on social media can help you own the challenge and motivate you to do more. I post pictures of myself working out all the time on Instagram and am so inspired by the feedback I receive.

5

Less Meat, More Plants

My Story

I've always been intrigued by vegetarians, vegans, pescatarians, and anyone who doesn't eat meat for one reason or another. As a physician, I know the research showing that a plant-based diet can significantly lower the risk of heart disease and colon and breast cancers. But on a personal level, I'm curious about how and why people choose to go meat-free.

My diet has always been fairly well rounded, but I do eat animal protein at just about every meal: eggs and bacon for breakfast, chicken Parmesan or grilled salmon over salad for lunch, and sushi, pork, or a bunless burger with a side salad for dinner. This menu, I realized last year, didn't include a variety of vegetables, fruits, beans, and other plants, which supply the range of nutrients and antioxidants we need for optimal health. In short, all I really ate were salad vegetables, with little exposure to broccoli, beets, Brussels sprouts, citrus fruits, sweet potatoes, kidney beans, kale, chia, edamame—you get the point.

When I told Chloe that I was thinking about going meat-free for my next challenge, she basically freaked out, telling me if I gave up meat completely without a solid plan in place, I'd lose muscle and possibly end up gaining fat by replacing protein with too many carbs. Or she said I wouldn't get enough protein and would wind up losing weight. Neither option seemed ideal! I knew she was right: I would have to create a specific daily meal plan that featured enough complete protein from vegetarian sources and follow it fairly rigidly. And while the idea appealed to me, the practicality didn't—it seemed like too much effort to be the kind of small change to my daily habits that I hoped to make during my challenge year.

So I decided that I would eliminate the worst animal protein in my diet: red meat, which science shows can increase cancer risk. This wouldn't be an easy feat for me: red meat is a large part of my diet, and two of my favorite foods to order out, which I do often living in New York City, are short ribs and carne asada—you'd understand the latter obsession if you ever ordered from my favorite Mexican restaurant down the street. At the same time, I vowed to eat more plants and focus on consuming a wider variety of fruits, veggies, and legumes.

Before the month began, I was anxious about the change. I haven't made many dietary tweaks in my life, so any meal modification was a big deal to me. Animal protein, especially red meat, also feels more filling than plant foods, so I was nervous about my appetite levels increasing over the next month. At the same time, I was excited to try something new. Similar to how I felt before my dry month and Push-ups and Planks Challenge, the idea of going outside my comfort zone for the betterment of my body was enough to make me eager for the month to start.

How to Get Over the Deprivation of Dropping a Food Group from Your Diet

Day 1 started with my typical eggs for breakfast and grilled chicken with a green salad for lunch—I know, not exactly re-creating the wheel here. But I didn't want to overhaul my daily diet by eating acai bowls or kale croquettes and getting turned off from the challenge before I had even begun.

That night, I was in Boston to visit friends, and we went to Legal Sea Foods for dinner. I sat down, opened the menu, and shazam—braised short ribs were on the menu. Despite the glaring fact we were at an establishment world renowned for its seafood, I needed those ribs. Their presence on the menu suddenly created an acute psychological stressor for me: the fact that I couldn't have my favorite meal made me want it all that much more. Part of this was due to the fact I had never expected to discover the dish on the menu that night. Had I known it would be there, like I had known there would be alcohol on the menu at every bar and restaurant in New York City during my Dry Challenge, I could have mentally prepared. Instead, I now took a deep breath and ordered lobster with sushi, with no attempt to find a new vegetable on the menu—it was painful enough to forgo the ribs; I didn't need to add insult to injury by getting some crazy Swiss chard salad that I might not enjoy.

The next few days were easier, though—no glaring temptations on any restaurant menus presented themselves to cause me a mini freak-out. But I noticed that I was already engaging in that powerful psychological dialogue between myself and my logic that I had during the Push-ups and Planks Challenge, rationalizing the reasons to stay on track toward my monthly goal. I kept reminding myself I couldn't eat red meat and that denial felt like deprivation, making me crave it that much more. When I went out to dinner again later that week and saw filet mignon on the menu, I felt I had to have it. I knew this was just my own mental insanity, though: I rarely ever ordered filet mignon! I might have found it funny the way our brains play games with our perceived preferences if I wasn't the victim of my own mind's toying.

After several days, though, I began to get over the deprivation by focusing instead on what I could eat—more plants. At the same time, the vegetarian gods decided to deliver me a blessing from above: I discovered online a food-delivery service called Daily Harvest, which sells organic, plant-based entrées, drinks, and soups. This was everything I was looking for: the food looked delicious, the entrées were reasonably priced, there were no added sugars or processed junk, they were easy and fast to make (hello, takeout alternative), and they could provide a greater variety of vegetables in my diet than I had had in years—things like kimchi, cauliflower, purple corn, green lentils, and chia. I ordered several soups and entrées for the following week. Now I had a plan in place to eat more plants.

Before my goodies arrived, I began to add more plants to my meals on my own, including berries with my eggs in the morning and ordering steamed veggies instead of salad for lunch. Nothing groundbreaking, but as you know from the push-ups and planks month, I'm a big believer in measured progression, and the additions made me feel like I was headed in the right direction.

At the week's end, I could tell my body was running cleaner—it was not a massive change, but I felt physically lighter, especially in and around my stomach. I also wasn't craving complex carbs, as I'd feared, especially since I was continuing to do more aerobic exercise after my Cardio Challenge. And I hadn't slipped up, either, but had overcome the initial deprivation that I was now learning seems to be part of all monthly challenges. By this point in the year, with several successful challenges under my belt, I knew some stress in the beginning was normal and if I could just get through the first few days, I'd be more focused and motivated for the rest of the month.

Week 2
How More Plants Can Lead to Less Body Fat

Get ready to be blown away by the diversity in my diet now . . . or not. I was now eating chicken nearly every day, which I don't particularly love, but without red meat, I felt I needed to double down on other animal proteins to prevent myself from wasting away. I knew this was a psychosomatic fear not based in fact, but regardless, I hadn't found a high-protein plant alternative or other type of animal meat that filled me up and I enjoyed as much as beef.

That changed midway through the week, though, after I stopped at a small market near my apartment on my way home from work. I was starving and while searching the shelves for something to sustain me, I saw smoked salmon—not part of my regular diet by any means. I bought it, and when I got home, I spread cream cheese on a piece, rolled it up, and devoured it. This was a concoction I'd never had before—and I loved it. It had more protein and healthy fats than chicken, not to mention it was tastier, more filling, and more convenient to pack for lunch or a snack. This was like discovering music while planking: it would help me take my challenge goals to a whole new level.

The next day, my Daily Harvest shipment arrived. I felt like a kid at Christmas unpacking frozen bowls of cauliflower kimchi, mushroom-carrot ginger soup, and lattes made from matcha and mushrooms with cacao. I brought the soup to work the next day and Christmas became New Year's Eve—it was fantastic and filling to boot. I've never particularly liked soup—it's never appealed to or satiated me. But Daily Harvest's mushroom-carrot ginger was fragrant, flavorful, and killed my appetite until it was time for dinner.

For the rest of the week, I took a soup to work every day for lunch. This was game-changing: not only was I now avoiding red meat, I wasn't eating animal meat at all and was consuming plant varieties I normally never would—foods like seaweed, reishi mushrooms, dulse, butternut squash, and spinach that were all in the soup. Some of these ingredients I had never even heard of before! I was even saving money by not ordering my standard chicken Parm. And the soup was lower in calories and higher in healthy fiber. This was truly Christmas (or Hanukkah) in May!

Later that week, I tried the cauliflower kimchi for dinner and it was just as fantastic—filling and flavorful. With these dishes, I wasn't even thinking about short ribs or burgers, let alone chicken, turkey, or pork. I felt like I now had a solid plan for the month and was excited to discover and try more new foods. And I was nailing the challenge goal of eating more plants, in a wider variety. Self-care never tasted so good!

While I was hesitant to accept there were negative consequences to my meat consumption, I was overjoyed when, at the end of Week 2, I'd lost a pound since the month's start. Weight loss had never been my goal, but just like during my Meditation and Cardio Challenges, it was certainly a nice side effect. I also felt less bloated and lighter on my feet.

Week 3
How to Lose the Dietary Bloat Without Missing Meat

Midway through the month, indiscretion finally struck one night when Chloe ordered takeout from our favorite Mexican restaurant. This is the place with the best carne asada in town, which we always order, as though we have some unstated mother-daughter pact. Whether it was a Freudian slip or Chloe truly forgot about my meat-free month, two orders of fragrant, spicy carne asada showed up at my door before I could remind her otherwise. I was screwed.

That's when I decided to make a deliberate decision to eat the beef. This wasn't a slip like on the mornings when I forgot to meditate or do planks and push-ups—this was 100 percent a conscious choice. Before digging my fork into the meat, I told myself I wasn't going to feel guilty about the decision, either, that this was an intentional slip of which I was fully aware. And the ominous part for my next two weeks was that the dish was delicious.

Immediately afterward, the scientist in me came out as I tried to discern if I felt any different or had those physical effects vegetarians and vegans talk about when they eat meat after months without. But I felt nothing, likely because I'd only been meat-free for a little over two weeks, which was hardly long enough to establish a new norm. As a scientist, I was disappointed not to see some side effects, but as a meat lover, I was pleased my foray into the red meat side hadn't been dark and disastrous.

To compensate for my slip, I had cauliflower kimchi for dinner the rest of the week, adding a scrambled egg to the dish to make it even more filling. With the egg, I figured I couldn't have any concerns, real or imagined, that I was short on protein because I wasn't eating meat.

This concoction caused me to realize something about my plant-based meals I hadn't before: my food was mushy. I barely had to chew anything! This was true of the soups, obviously, but also of my sautéed veggies, the veggie burgers I'd see my friends order, the tofu and bean-based dishes I saw online, and the grain bowls popular at restaurants across the city. These meals weren't like a steak or short ribs, where you have to chew for seconds just to be able to swallow. By comparison, a baby could have eaten my cauliflower kimchi (except for the spiciness, of course!).

Crunching and chewing are satisfying sensations, though, and I decided to make up for the missing mastication so I didn't crave meat simply because I wasn't chewing as much. For this reason alone, I bought carrot and celery sticks and started having them with my kimchi or with hummus as an afternoon snack. Turns out, this small adaptation had big effects, giving me the mouth sensation of chewing I had started to miss.

By this time, there was no denying my stomach was significantly flatter. I'd lost weight but I was also noticeably less bloated. I had not expected these results in just a few weeks' time! And avoiding meat was certainly physically easier than all the aerobic exercise I'd done last month. But that's why I liked these monthly challenges: there was always self-discovery in each and every one. I never knew or could anticipate how a change would affect me—physically, mentally, or emotionally—until I adopted it for a few weeks. And so far, I really liked the effects of less meat and more plants.

Week 4
How to Retrain Your Brain to Make Healthier Decisions

Finally, I was in the homestretch, but not in the clear, as I learned early in the week. I was dining out at my favorite Mexican restaurant when the waiter took my order and, out of habit, I asked for the carne asada. (I know by now you are probably questioning why I seem to be addicted to this one Mexican dish!)

I stopped myself midsentence, ordering instead some octopus tacos and a quesadilla with zucchini flowers—you've got to appreciate the culinary variety in New York City. Nevertheless, I was disturbed by how my brain seemed to continually function on autopilot. Was I so programmed that I ordered only out of habit? After all, I'd asked for a menu and even looked at it, yet here I was, spitting out the same order I had already told myself I wouldn't get.

This was a fascinating realization for me as a scientist interested in human behavior. Do we ever really make conscious decisions about what we eat and drink? Or are our preferences trained by habit? How many daily lifestyle decisions do we make mindlessly, without even thinking? And why? Is it because we're always in a rush? Or are our brains just so overloaded with outer and inner distractions that we don't have time to think and choose? Is it possible to retrain our brains to make healthier choices based on self-will and true desire, not habit? Yes, these are the kinds of things I think about after a good Mexican meal!

This was an interesting epiphany—but one that didn't prevent me from making an actual slip later in the week. With only two days remaining in the month, I ordered meatballs at a restaurant—and once again, the decision was deliberate.

I was traveling and eating at a steakhouse—not my choice—where there was a delicious-sounding meatball appetizer on the menu. I weighed the decision, tried to consider other menu items, and then told myself I had only two days left in the challenge and it wouldn't change my experiment whether I had meatballs now or forty-eight hours later. I also justified it by promising to continue the challenge into the next month. This was how good my brain was at rationalizing the things I wanted.

Despite my fourth-quarter slip, my results at the end of the month were amazing. I was still lighter on the scale, but more important, I felt healthier and had zero bloat. Giving up red meat had been less of a hardship than I expected and I'd found flavorful, filling, and more nutritious foods that I knew would be part of my diet going forward. In fact, just like I had been at the end of my dry month, I was excited to continue the challenge into June. My epiphany in the Mexican restaurant helped me to realize I could make conscious decisions about what I ate, that I didn't need to be programmed by habit. And the more deliberate decisions I made to eat healthy, the more those choices would become automatic. Over time, healthier decisions can become habits if we let them.

MAY LESS MEAT, MORE PLANTS:
The Science Behind Eating Less Meat, More Plants

Red meat, or beef, lamb, pork, and veal, isn't unhealthy in moderation. It's high in protein; rich in heme iron (which the body absorbs better than the iron in plants); and a good source of B vitamins, selenium, and zinc. Although pricey, organic, grass-fed beef is also rich in healthy fats, making it, along with its protein, one of the most satiating foods you can eat calorie for calorie. Despite these attributes, though, science has found that eating too much red meat can raise the risk of certain diseases—and Americans are eating too much of it. At the same time, we're not consuming enough plants, mainly fruits and vegetables: according to the Centers for Disease Control and Prevention (CDC), 90 percent of Americans don't meet the daily recommendation to eat one and a half cups of fruits and two to three cups of vegetables. Reducing how much meat you consume and making more room for plants in your diet is not restrictive—there are, after all, far more varieties of plant foods than red meat, considered a luxury in most countries. Here's how simply switching the focus of what you eat can help you get healthier and leaner.

The Frightening Link Between Red Meat and Breast Cancer

While the science isn't conclusive, researchers have found a link between red meat and breast cancer. Perhaps the strongest evidence comes from the U.S. Nurses' Health Study II, one of the largest research efforts to date on how diet affects disease. The study found women who consumed one and a half servings of red meat daily had a 22 percent greater chance of developing breast cancer than those who ate red meat only once per week. Similarly, a separate study from researchers at the Harvard School of Public Health discovered the more red meat women eat as teens and young adults, the greater their risk of developing breast cancer later on in life.

The reasons red meat is thought to be associated with an increased breast cancer risk are numerous and complex. Conventional grain-fed beef contains hormones and other chemicals associated with breast cancer, while researchers also blame carcinogens that form on beef and pork during high-heat cooking like grilling, smoking, and barbecuing. Nitrates, or chemicals found in processed meats like sausage, bacon, hot dogs, salami, and ham, also boost cancer risk, so much so that the World Health Organization now lists these foods as probable human carcinogens.

Eating Too Much Red Meat Can Lead to Colon Cancer

While the association between red meat and breast cancer isn't concrete, the link between colon cancer and consuming beef and pork is. Large, long-term studies show that the more red meat people consume, the greater their risk of developing the disease. In fact, a study conducted by the World Health Organization found that eating fifty grams of processed red meat per day—less than two slices of bacon—raises colon cancer risk by 18 percent.

Red Meat Can Increase Your Risk of Death from Any Cause

According to a 2017 study of more than a half-million Americans published in *BMJ,* those who eat the most red meat are 26 percent more likely to die from eight different diseases, including stroke, heart disease, and diabetes, than those who consume less. The reasons red meat are considered by some to be deadly are manifold. When it comes to heart disease and stroke, scientists say red meat contains an amino acid that our intestines turn into a compound that speeds artery hardening. Researchers also say some people may even be allergic to meat, a condition that results in the creation of more arterial plaque.

Avoiding Red Meat Is One of the Best Ways to Beat Bloat

If you're eating more red meat on a low-carb or ketogenic diet and not seeing results you want, blame the beef. Red meat takes longer to digest than almost all other foods, which can lead to bloating, gas, and constipation. That's not all: beef, pork, and lamb may also disrupt the balance of healthy bacteria in our guts, which can cause a host of gastrointestinal problems. For example, a 2017 study published in the journal *Gut* found people who eat the most red meat are 58 percent more likely to develop diverticulitis, a painful bowel condition. Conversely, eating less meat and more plant-based foods has been shown to increase digestion and prevent GI issues.

Eating More Plants Will Boost Your Metabolism, Skin Health, and Brain Function

An overwhelming body of research shows that following a plant-based diet—whether you're vegetarian, vegan, or pescatarian or simply choose to eat mostly whole grains, vegetables, beans, nuts, seeds, and fruits—is one of the best ways to prevent chronic disease like cancer, heart disease, diabetes, arthritis, and Alzheimer's. Plants, in their whole form, may be just as potent as prescription drugs, working on a cellular level to reduce the systemic inflammation responsible for many health issues. Plants are higher in vitamins, minerals, fiber, antioxidants, and phytochemicals than other foods, calorie for calorie, and we absorb them more effectively through food than supplements or engineered foods like sports bars. For these reasons, consuming more plants has been shown to increase just about every physical function, including metabolism, digestion, cognitive function, and skin health.

Plants Are Powerful Antidepressants

There's a reason why studies show that people who eat the most plants report less depression, anxiety, stress, and mood disorders.

Whole vegetables, fruits, nuts, and beans are packed with antioxidants that go straight to the brain, helping to repair cellular damage and reduce inflammation, both of which can have a profound effect on mood. Moreover, plants contain antioxidants that work similarly to antidepressants, suppressing enzymes that can contribute to depression. Plants like leafy greens, broccoli, mushrooms, and soybeans are also great sources of the amino acid tryptophan, which the body needs to produce serotonin. Turkey also contains this amino acid—you've likely heard how it can make you sleepy on Thanksgiving—but the body better converts tryptophan from plants than animal meat. Plants' effects on well-being go beyond boosting serotonin and reducing the risk of depression and anxiety. Researchers have also found that those who eat more vegetables and fruits reported feeling more motivation, energy, and overall vitality.

Eating a Plant-Based Diet Can Help You Lose Weight Without Effort

When I started my Less Meat, More Plants Challenge, it wasn't my goal to lose weight. So I was pleasantly surprised when, after four weeks, I had lost a little fat without trying, and I felt lighter and leaner despite eating what I had wanted, barring red meat. This was counterintuitive, too, since I've always consumed animal meat, like diets recommend, to feel full and reduce carb cravings.

As it turns out, though, researchers have long known eating plants is an effective way to lose weight. Plant-based diets are naturally high in fiber and nutrients, yet low in calories, providing substantial nutrition that keeps you feeling full without the need to eliminate food groups or count calories or carbs. In this sense, plant-based eating doesn't feel restrictive or like a diet at all, adding to its success rate and sustainability. One 2018 study published in *The Journal of the American Medical Association* even found people could lose a significant amount of weight in one year simply by eating more whole grains, legumes, vegetables, and fruit, without counting calories or even restricting how much they eat. In part for this reason, science shows, on average, vegetarians are slimmer than their omnivore friends.

Don't Become a Plant-Food Junkie

Many vegetarians and vegans don't reap the benefits of a plant-based diet because they replace animal foods with meat- and dairy-free junk foods, made from processed grains and other harmful ingredients like enriched wheat flour, vegetable shortening, tapioca starch, and added sugars like brown rice syrup. While all these items are technically plant-based, they're highly processed, tend to be high in calories, and are not good sources of protein, fiber, antioxidants, vitamins, and the other nutrients that make plant-based foods so beneficial. For healthy plant-based eating, stick to whole or fresh foods that have had little done to them from earth to dinner table.

MAY LESS MEAT, MORE PLANTS: Your Story

Changing your diet isn't easy, especially if you try to make a massive overhaul and severely reduce how much you eat or eliminate an entire food group or more than one at a time. That's why several studies show that 90 to 95 percent of dieters end up regaining any weight they lost within months or even weeks of ending a massive nutritional overhaul. Reducing how much red meat you eat and consuming more plants, on the other hand, isn't a massive overhaul—exactly why I picked it to be a monthly challenge. Whether you eat meat every day or rarely consume animal protein, boosting your plant consumption for thirty days is a doable and sustainable goal. Here are ten ways to make a month of eating less meat and more plants work for you.

1. INDIVIDUALIZE THE CHALLENGE. If you currently eat red meat twice a day, it may be difficult for you to give it up entirely. I would encourage you to try, but the end goal of this month is to reduce how much red meat you eat while increasing your intake of vegetables, beans, fruit, and other plants. With that in mind, devise a challenge you know you can sustain for thirty days without resorting to junk food— that is, don't swap your nightly steak for fried chicken—or sacrificing on the intent to eat more plants, which is just as important a part of this month as eating less red meat.

   If you don't eat any red meat, consider cutting back on chicken, turkey, and other animal proteins, while if you're a pescatarian, vegetarian, or vegan, forgoing red meat, use this month to try to eat healthier whole or fresh plant foods. Before you begin, analyze your daily diet and see where you can swap out processed items like crackers, pasta, bread, snack foods, vegan cheeses, and meatless alternatives for healthier whole foods.

2. PLAN AHEAD. Our food choices aren't ingrained only in our brains but also in our daily routines, restaurants, and refrigerators. If you routinely eat steak and burgers at home, dine out on restaurant meat-heavy meals, and/or your kitchen is full of frozen patties, hot dogs, pork chops, and bacon, it'll be difficult to be successful this month. Before the challenge begins, do some online surfing for healthier meal ideas you can easily make at home or bring for breakfast, lunch, and dinner. Find new restaurants, takeout options, or home-delivery services that offer plant-based entrées you'd like to try. Finally, restock your kitchen with fish, turkey, chicken,

and other beef- and pork-free proteins, along with fresh vegetables, fruits, beans, and whole grains.

3. FOCUS ON ADDING, NOT ELIMINATING. Continually remind-
    ing myself that I was adding a large number of foods to my
    diet, not just eliminating red meat, made this challenge
    immensely easier. While I spent the first few days fixated
    on the fact I was depriving myself of short ribs and carne
    asada, this fixation went away as soon as I realized there
    were dozens of new and exciting foods I could and should
    be eating. So instead of focusing on what you can't have—
    beef, lamb, pork, and veal—think about all the foods you can
    eat, including delicious items like sweet potatoes, quinoa,
    black beans, cashews, seaweed salad, roasted corn, water-
    melon, nectarines . . . The list is literally endless.

4. FIND ALTERNATIVES THAT PROVIDE THE SAME PROTEIN,
    SATISFACTION, OR CHEWING SENSATION AS RED MEAT. This
    is a great chance to discover new foods you might enjoy even
    more than red meat—and that are healthier to boot. For me,
    my great discovery was smoked salmon with cream cheese,
    which was just as satisfying and high in protein as short
    ribs, but with more healthy fats and nutrients I don't nor-
    mally eat and without the negative health effects associated
    with red meat. The Daily Harvest deliveries allowed me to
    boost my vegetable intake in ways I couldn't imagine while
    working so well with my on-the-go lifestyle. (If you opt for a
    home-delivery food service, just be sure the ingredients are
    primarily whole foods, not processed ingredients or added
    sugars.)
        You may also want to find something that gives you the
    same mouth sensation as meat. When I started eating
    more cooked vegetables, I missed chewing food. That went
    away as soon as I started eating carrot and celery sticks

with hummus. You might prefer the crunchiness of nuts or seeds, which make great meat alternatives since they're also high in protein and healthy fats. Other healthy, chewable plant-based options include crudité with cottage or cream cheese, dried peas, roasted chickpeas, kale chips, and air-popped popcorn.

5.   DON'T JUST FOCUS ON THE SCALE. If you're successful at this month's challenge, swapping out calorie-dense meats and processed carbs for more whole plants will likely cause you to lose weight. But don't allow yourself to get fixated on the scale. Weight loss takes time, and for any dietary change to be sustainable and trigger the lasting weight loss you want, it's more important to pay attention to how your body feels than what the scale tells you. When you focus on eating more plants and less red meat and processed foods, you should have more energy, improved digestion, and even better bowel movements. But not all plant foods produce the same effects on everyone. Pay attention to what you eat and try to discern which foods make you feel good and which ones slow you down. Ultimately, the foods that make you feel good are the foods you should prioritize in your diet.

6.   BE OPEN TO TRYING NEW OR EXOTIC FOODS. Part of what made this month so fun for me was trying foods I hadn't had before or eaten in years. There are hundreds of different vegetables, fruits, beans, and nuts and seeds, along with many ways of preparing them—don't close yourself off to trying them based on old assumptions or one negative experience. Our taste buds change, as do the way foods are commonly prepared. Use this month to expand your culinary experience and expertise.

I also found it helpful to consider new categories of food. For example, I've never been particularly fond of soup, but for the month's challenge, the vegetable soups from Daily Harvest became a satisfying and important part of my diet. They were low in calories, yet still filling, which I know contributed to my flatter stomach by the month's end.

7. LOOK ONLINE FOR CREATIVE PLANT-BASED RECIPES. There are a ton of interesting, tasty, and innovative meat-free recipes online, oftentimes posted by bloggers. These Internet chefs now influence the culinary world at large, inspiring new trends like swapping cauliflower for potatoes, flour, and rice in traditional recipes and making avocados the star of nearly every conceivable dish. Looking for a new spin on a favorite dish made with red meat or animal protein? You can likely find through online research a plant-based version that is just as flavorful if not more so than the traditional recipe.

8. EAT BREAKFAST FOR DINNER. Adding an egg to my nightly cauliflower kimchi turned the vegan meal into a protein-packed dinner. Eggs pack a whopping seven grams of complete protein in only seventy-five calories, making them one of the most protein-rich foods per calorie. Eggs are also a good source of healthy fat, which will help you stay full when you're not eating meat. Yet despite these attributes, Americans often think of eggs only for breakfast when the ingredient works just as well for lunch or dinner. Think of new items like vegetable frittatas; egg tacos; egg bakes; tomato or spinach shakshuka; or dinner omelets with cheese, herbs, and veggies.

9. FIND SNEAKY, SATISFYING WAYS TO ADD VEGETABLES TO YOUR DIET. One great benefit to the low-carb trend is that it's forced chefs and food bloggers to find new ways to make pasta, bread, and other high-carb favorites using lower-carb, lower-calorie plants. Many restaurants, fast-casual chains,

and food-delivery companies now offer pasta dishes made from zucchini, beet, or carrot noodles—you can also make these veggie "zoodles" yourself by looking for recipes on-line. Similarly, mashed and minced cauliflower has become a popular alternative to mashed potatoes and regular rice. Cauliflower is even now used as a meat substitute, served as "steak" when grilled or roasted and with buffalo sauce in lieu of chicken wings. If you have a sweet tooth, try ice cream or crepes made from banana or banana and eggs or swap mashed black beans or avocado for oil in brownie and cake recipes.

10. USE THE MONEY YOU'RE SAVING ON MEAT FOR FRESH, SEA-SONAL FRUITS AND VEGETABLES. One reason Americans don't eat as many fruits and veggies as those in other coun-tries is that we don't prioritize fresh, seasonal produce. But the kind of fruits and veggies we buy is critical to our enjoyment of these foods. For example, would you enjoy a peach that's juicy and ripe—or one that's mealy, mushy, or not ripe because it has sat on a truck for days or been grown with so many chemicals? Many conventional farm-ers grow produce for size, ability to withstand travel, and aesthetic quality, not flavor or nutritional quality. All this can make fruits and veggies, especially those that are out of season and imported from faraway places, taste flavor-less and bland. Use the money you'd save on meat and put it toward buying organic, seasonal fruits and vegetables that are grown locally or at least within the regional area. You may be pleasantly surprised by how much better these foods taste when they haven't been shipped from far away or grown solely for visual appeal.

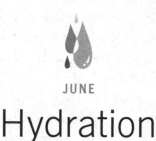

6

JUNE

Hydration

My Story

I've had three kidney stones in my lifetime. While these excruciating little babies can be caused by many things, including diet, prescription drugs, and hormone imbalances, in my case, each and every one was due to dehydration.

I don't care what you hear: kidney stones are ten times more painful than giving birth. One of my stones required a stent, which meant a trip to the operating room to go under anesthesia. Not only was all this unpleasant, it was also dangerous.

Dehydration, even a mild case, doesn't just cause kidney stones. It also ages your skin; interferes with proper heart, brain, and liver function; and makes your blood thicker and more viscous. Dehydration can cause headaches, nausea, bad breath, fatigue, weight gain, confusion, and even seizures.

As a doctor, I know better than to let myself get dehydrated. But as a working professional with a busy schedule, regular hydration has somehow never been top of mind between med school, raising children, and now juggling a full-time television career with a booming medical practice. There are many days when I've woken up at 5 A.M. and by dinnertime, all I've had are several cups of coffee, possibly with a glass of tequila after work. Yes, that's right: zero water consumption other than what I get through food. And the only reason I don't hydrate is out of pure laziness: I either forget or don't want to have to take the time to use the bathroom, which is the lamest excuse ever, but the truth.

When I began taking stock of how to improve my health this year, drinking more water was an easy choice for a challenge. I knew it was a daily oversight that was impacting my health and happiness, and from my current continual state of mild dehydration, I had nowhere to go but up.

Yet figuring out exactly how much water to drink daily wasn't easy, despite my access to all the best medical experts and research. Yes, you've likely heard the recommendation to drink eight ounces of water eight times per day, but turns out, that's somewhat of a wellness legend. No large medical institution has ever conducted a solid large-scale study of how much water we need to drink every day, in part because hydration needs are distinctly individual, based on your body size, activity level, sweat rate, and how much water you consume through food.

Before beginning the month, I studied all the science I could find on the topic before settling on the hydration recommendation made by the Institute of Medicine (now called the National Academy of Medicine), which advises women consume approximately 2.7 liters (90 ounces) of water a day from beverages and food, with men consuming approximately 3.7 liters (125 ounces). I decided not to factor water from food as it's nearly impossible to calculate, even for a science dork like me. And about 80 percent of our hydration comes from the water and other beverages we drink, anyway.

With this in mind, I went out and bought three 800-milliliter (27-ounce) glass water bottles. My plan was to fill each with filtered water, then drink all three by the end of the day, giving myself 2.4 liters (81 ounces) of water total for the day. While this was still 0.3 liters shy of the IOM's daily recommendation, I'd make up the rest with coffee and food. And it'd be a giant improvement over the near-zero liters of water I was currently drinking.

As part of the challenge, I decided only water and seltzer would count toward my daily hydration goal—not soda, diet soda, juice, alcohol, or other beverages that contain sugar or other additives. Plus, five months after nailing January's Dry Challenge, I was still adamant about consuming less booze and making sure I didn't exceed seven actual servings of alcohol per week. Counting a tequila cocktail toward my daily hydration goal now would be not only insane but inaccurate, since alcohol in itself is dehydrating, as anyone

Why Drink Only Water This Month?

Simply put, water is the most effective way to hydrate your body. Not only do soda and juice contain sugar and calories, which aren't good for your overall health, they are also difficult for your stomach to digest, which can aggravate dehydration. Sports drinks are also high in sugar, making them unnecessary unless you're exercising vigorously or for hours on end. As for diet soda, most contain artificial sweeteners and other unhealthy additives. I've always remembered this story a friend told me who interviewed Melissa Etheridge shortly after the singer was diagnosed with breast cancer. My friend was drinking diet soda during the interview when Etheridge told her that she should stop. After my friend balked, Etheridge suggested my friend do an experiment with two house plants: feed one plant only water for six months and the other only diet soda and see which plant does better. After all, as Etheridge pointed out to my friend, our bodies are made up of 60 percent water, not 60 percent diet soda.

who's ever had too much to drink knows. In addition, I didn't want to try to adopt a new habit that includes unhealthy components, which soda and juice are in excess.

Just a Few Days of Drinking More Water Can Up Your Energy Levels

What was fantastic about this challenge was that I already had a game plan in place before the month began: all I had to do was follow it. The night before, I filled my three 800-milliliter bottles with filtered water and stuck them in the fridge so they'd be chilled and ready to go in the morning. When I woke up at 5 A.M. the next day, I grabbed two bottles—one to drink at *GMA* and the other to sip while at my medical office—and headed out the door. While in the taxi to the studio, I started sipping on the first bottle. What this meant, I realized, was that by 5:30 A.M. on my first day of the challenge, I had already consumed more water than I normally would. Nailing it out of the gate!

That morning, I announced with Robin Roberts on air that we would both be doing a Hydration Challenge for the month. We wanted to drive home to viewers that subsisting on a less-than-optimal amount of water can harm your health in ways most people never think about, like causing you to look older and even gain weight!

When I left *GMA*, I had finished the first bottle, which was fairly easy for me to do while sitting through hair and makeup and waiting on set. But the second bottle was another story.

My schedule is so jammed when I'm at my practice that I usually don't have time to sit, let alone eat lunch, go to the bathroom, make a phone call, or even return my kids' texts. I see patients back to back, and I like to spend as much time with each one as possible while giving them my full attention—stopping to drink from a water bottle when they're discussing their personal health problems seemed rude.

When I'm finished seeing patients for the day, there's always paperwork to complete, conversations to have with my staff about patient care, and scheduling issues to work out. I was also concerned that if I drank too much, I'd keep patients waiting because I'd continually be running to the bathroom. Yes, you would think I wouldn't be so crazed that I couldn't even make time to go to the ladies' room—and I was trying to keep up my meditation practice to help stay more zen about time management—but when I'm at work, I feel like I'm on a go-go-go treadmill. Stepping off for a minute might shake up the entire race. For these reasons, on Day 1, I was barely able to take a few sips from the bottle in my office refrigerator, never mind drink the whole thing.

Thankfully, the third bottle was waiting chilled at home for me. I pulled it out as soon as I stepped in the door and started sipping while changing out of my clothes. I finished the full bottle within an hour, in part to make up for the hydration I'd missed during the day, but also because I was worried if I didn't drink it by 9 P.M., I'd be up all night in the bathroom.

The rest of the week followed suit as the first day. I continued to nail the morning bottle, struggled with the afternoon one, and usually finished my nightcap. Although I was falling short of my 2.4-liter daily target, I was pleased I was consuming nearly triple the water that I had before the challenge started.

As the week went on—and throughout the rest of the month—I began to experiment with the taste and temperature of water. I knew that if I made hydration as palatable as possible, I'd be able to keep it up more easily. I tried water with ice, without ice, at room temperature, and with lemon, lime, and even cucumber and orange slices like I'd seen at the spa. I felt like I was on a mindful journey to find my ideal taste and temperature. In the end, I decided I just like cold water, no fruit or ice. And while I would have never thought it before, arriving at this simple conclusion made the challenge feel more fun, like a culinary experiment.

At the end of the week, I knew I'd picked a rock-star challenge for me. Increasing my water intake was already benefiting my health in quantifiable ways, which I could tell by the color of my urine. (Don't be grossed out—examining pee is a great way to assess your health, which is why physicians are so enthusiastic about getting you to pee in one of those tiny cups.) Normally dark and concentrated, my pee was now a pale yellow—a sign my body was finally hydrated enough to function better. After a week of more water, I also felt more energetic, less irritable, and even more sated by my meals. And while I was still having difficulty getting that second bottle down at work, I was consuming at least two more liters of water per day than I normally did. Oh, and all those trips to the bathroom I'd been so worried about? While I may have had to make one or two additional trips throughout the day, the inconvenience was much less than I had imagined.

Week 2

How Drinking More Water Doused My Afternoon Appetite

Before my Hydration Challenge, my morning routine included four cups of coffee, consumed between 5 A.M. and noon nearly every day. But now, as I began Week 2, I noticed I was drinking less coffee because I wasn't so dependent on the minor hydration it provides. This reinforced what I've recognized as a physician, but rarely applied to myself: It's not just what you eat and drink but also what you don't eat and drink. In other words, my dietary choices were having an inverse impact on my consumption or lack thereof of other foods and beverages. The more water I drank, the less coffee I had. The same was true during my dry month, although for slightly different reasons: since I didn't consume any alcohol, I ended up drinking more water and seltzer because they were the healthiest substitutes to order in bars and restaurants.

Trying to get to that second bottle at work still wasn't going well, though, and I knew I needed a different strategy. I decided I'd be more comfortable drinking in front of patients if I did so out of a glass rather than a bottle, which would be easy enough to do since we offer sparkling water in glasses in the waiting room. So I began treating myself like a patient, taking a glass of sparkling into appointments with me. With this approach, I kicked up my daytime consumption by at least a glass and a half, or to about 350 milliliters.

At the end of the second week, I noticed a profound change in my hunger. While I'd felt slightly more sated with my meals at the end of Week 1, I was now perceptibly fuller and never got that growling sensation in my stomach I often do in the late afternoons. I wasn't eating less per se, but I was less ravenous, which meant I was able to make healthier choices about what I wanted to eat rather than just finding anything to put in my stomach.

Week 3
Forget Serums: This Is the Secret to Younger Skin

Midway through the month, I already felt I had made hydration a new habit. It was now routine for me to wake up at 5 A.M., meditate, try to get in some push-ups and planks, and then grab my first water bottle to sip on the way to the studio. I was still drinking less coffee, but oddly had more energy. I just felt like my engine was running cleaner, which is hardly a medical assessment, but the best way I can describe knowing I was now regularly flushing toxins and metabolic buildup out of my kidneys and other organs.

My urine was also paler than what I had first noticed earlier in the month, and I could tell my digestion was improving now that my stomach had water to process food with. My appetite was still far lower than it had been in previous months, abolishing any hollow-pit hunger feelings.

As for work, things were better there, too, as I continued to drink up to a solid two glasses of sparkling water. I now used my second water bottle to drink from while I was in the car going to my practice, using all the free time I could find to hydrate.

At the end of the week, I had a happy surprise: my skin was starting to look drastically better, even more so than during my Dry Challenge in January. This wasn't a shock per se—at the beginning of the month, I had said on *GMA* how essential hydration is to skin health—but I was amazed to see it firsthand. Here I was, willing to spend tons of money on fancy face creams and antiaging products, and this one simple and inexpensive change had produced better results, leaving my skin plumper and more hydrated.

Week 4

Turning a Simple New Health Habit into Sustained Success

The last week of the challenge, I started to experience something I never had before: my mouth was moist. Okay, I can totally see how this may seem like an odd discovery to some, but as a person who constantly notices a dry mouth sensation, causing me to want to brush my teeth or have a mint or gum after every meal, this was a wonderful revelation. As it turns out, not drinking enough water kills your saliva production, allowing bacteria to grow, which can lead to bad breath. Now, though, my mouth felt healthier, my teeth were cleaner, and I didn't feel like I needed gum after meals, no matter what I ate, even if it was pungent or garlicky. My tongue also looked glistening and moist, not pasty and dry, which, according to both traditional and Eastern medicine, meant my overall health was good.

Similar to the last few weeks, I continued to drink less coffee but had more energy. Since I was now never ravenous, I was eating healthier—keeping up May's challenge to eat more plants and less red meat was easier because I felt fuller and more satisfied after meals, even if they didn't include a whopping portion of animal protein. My skin continued to appear even more hydrated as the days went on, and the tone had also started to improve. I had nearly obviated the annoying need to brush or chew gum after every meal, and I hadn't had to go to the bathroom nearly as often as I'd imagined. Why hadn't I started drinking water before this month?!

I couldn't believe how much such a simple tweak had affected how I felt, looked, ate, and lived. And I hadn't even realized that I had been doing anything to hurt my health by failing to consume enough water on a daily basis. After all, except for the kidney stones, I didn't see any drastic effects from my mild dehydration. But now I realized that without drinking enough water before this month, I had been able to live, but I wasn't living optimally. The change was small and didn't take a huge effort—this wasn't like motivating myself to go to the gym or a SoulCycle class—but the results were eye-opening and potentially life-changing.

After the month ended, I didn't change my morning routine: I still grabbed a water bottle before leaving my apartment in the morning. I continued to sip sparkling water in my office and finished a full water bottle at night, too. When I don't follow this routine, it's like missing a morning of meditation—it leaves a hole in my day. I'm noticeably crankier, hungrier, and more sluggish, and my whole body just feels dry, especially my skin.

Several months later, I stopped at a market near my apartment where I've been shopping for months. The woman behind the counter, whom I've seen nearly every day for the last two years, looked at me oddly, then stopped me as she was ringing up my items to tell me that I had amazing skin—something neither she nor anyone else had ever said to me before. Nothing had changed about my routine that would have affected my skin in that way except that I had been drinking more water for several months. I thanked her and left, knowing that this one small wellness tweak was going to have ramifications for years to come.

JUNE HYDRATION:
The Science Behind Optimal Hydration

Three-Quarters of All Americans Are Chronically Dehydrated

Think you drink enough? You probably don't. A survey of more than three thousand Americans conducted by researchers at New York–Presbyterian/Weill Cornell Medical Center found that as many as 75 percent of us don't meet the IOM's hydration recommendation, meaning most of us are clinically and chronically dehydrated. Bottled water is the United States's best-selling beverage, but the most popular size is just a scant 0.5 liters—2.2 liters shy of the daily recommendation for women and 3.2 liters below the daily recommendation for men. And our next choices for beverages—soda, coffee, and beer—can all act like a diuretic on the body.

I see this in my own practice, where the majority of urine samples we take from patients come back too dark and concentrated. When I share with them that they're dehydrated and it's making their symptoms or medical issues worse, they often agree and promise to start drinking more. But year after year, I see the same patients—and the same dark urine samples and health complications from chronic dehydration.

Try Water Before Popping a Pill for Headaches

Our bodies may be made up of 60 percent water, but our brains, composed of 73 percent water, need even more. What happens when you don't drink enough water is that your brain can begin to physically shrink, contracting slightly from your skull, which causes a headache that can range from mild to full-on migraine. Dehydration also causes blood vessels to narrow, which can increase the severity of any pain.

You don't have to be clinically dehydrated to get a headache, either: even mild dehydration can bring on head pain. By the time you feel any pain, it's usually too late to prevent a headache. But if you suffer from frequent headaches, try drinking more throughout the day and week. Chances are, you'll be surprised by the effect.

Water Can Trigger Weight Loss in More Ways Than One

What you drink can widen your waistline. Soda, juice, sugary smoothies, fancy coffee drinks, and cocktails are all high in sugar and calories, and low in healthy fat, protein, and fiber, causing insulin levels to spike and your body to store fat.

But what you *don't* drink can also do damage to your waistline. Not consuming enough water can increase appetite and affect your body's metabolic function, hormone levels, and ability to exercise and control cravings. Part of the problem is that the same area of your brain that controls appetite also controls thirst. When you're dehydrated, that area of your brain goes into overload, sending signals that may cause you to want to reach for a bagel when what you really need is a water bottle.

Drinking water and staying hydrated also helps fill your stomach, increasing feelings of fullness. Try it yourself the next time you're ravenous by drinking two eight-ounce glasses of water in a matter of minutes. Most likely, your hunger will be abated, if not eliminated.

Surprisingly, dehydration can interfere with a healthy metabolism. According to several studies, even mild dehydration may slow the body's ability to burn calories. At the same time, one 2003 report published in *The Journal of Clinical Endocrinology & Metabolism* found that drinking more water, regardless of how hydrated you are, can bump up your metabolism temporarily by as much as 30 percent. Drinking ice water has an even bigger metabolic boost, as your system works to warm the beverage to body temperature. It's basic thermodynamics!

Hydration also aids in digestion—one reason why nutritionists recommend drinking water with every meal. I used to never drink water with food, but now I can't imagine eating without it. Finally, if you're dehydrated, it can be difficult to summon the physical and mental energy you need to exercise or even move more during everyday activities.

Dehydration May Be as Detrimental to Your Heart as Smoking

While we have heard plenty about how eating poorly, being over-weight, having a family history, and even being exposed to pollution can increase the risk of heart disease, we almost never hear about a common yet extremely preventable cause: dehydration. Chronic dehydration, which most Americans suffer from, decreases blood volume while constricting the diameter of arteries and veins, both of which cause the heart to work harder to pump blood throughout the body. This, in turn, can increase blood pressure and heart rate, which can boost the risk of palpitation, blood clots, deep vein thrombosis, and stroke. Studies show nearly half of all people who suffer a stroke are dehydrated, while heart attacks are most likely to occur after people wake up in the morning, when they're most likely to be dehydrated. In fact, recent research finds that mild dehydration can impair heart function nearly as much as one cigarette, according to the 2016 study published in the *European Journal of Nutrition*. For these reasons, staying properly hydrated can decrease the risk of coronary heart disease by as much as 59 percent in women and 46 percent in men, according to research.

Water Is One of the Best and Least Expensive Antiaging Remedies

I now know from personal experience the powerful effect that simple hydration can have on your skin. I'd never had such youthful, plump, and even-toned skin as I did after a few weeks of drinking more water. And it's not just me: A 2015 study published in *Clinical, Cosmetic and Investigational Dermatology* shows that staying hydrated boosts the water content of cells in both the deep and superficial layers of your skin's epidermis. This increases skin elasticity and works to prevent and even reverse fine lines and blotchiness. Not drinking enough water, on the other hand, limits the body's ability to flush toxins that accumulate in skin cells, increasing the appearance of premature aging, along with skin conditions like eczema, psoriasis, and discoloration.

Hydration Prevents and Treats Urinary Tract Infections

We have a saying in surgery: *The best antidote to pollution is dilution.* What this means is that after gloves, tools, and blood have been inside an open wound or incision, a surgeon has to irrigate the site with water before closing the skin—otherwise, the risk of infection increases. In other words, you have to get rid of the pollution with dilution or the pollution will cause problems. I tell this to all my patients who have urinary tract infections, which a good percentage of my practice has—the painful condition affects nearly half of all women. Not only can dehydration trigger UTIs, but not drinking enough can also prevent your body from being able to clear the infection.

Dehydration Can Make You Tired, Cranky, and Sluggish

During the month's challenge, I discovered that when I'm hydrated, I have more energy and patience and take more pleasure in all life's little—and not so little—moments. Turns out, hydration's effect on mood is well supported by science. Studies show that even mild dehydration can lead to lethargy, irritability, and fatigue and cause you to perceive tasks as more difficult. You may also have trouble concentrating when you're dehydrated and even be more susceptible to anger and mood swings.

Water Will Make You Smarter

Since our brains are made up of 73 percent water, it's not surprising that proper hydration helps boost cognitive function. In fact, drinking eight to ten cups of water can amplify your brain's ability to think and work by as much as 30 percent, studies show. Meanwhile, 2014 research published in the American College of Sports Medicine's *Health & Fitness Journal* has also found that subsisting at just a 1 percent hydration deficit can interfere with your ability to think. That's not all: proper hydration also increases the brain's ability to concentrate and retain information—one reason why even a case of mild dehydration can trigger short-term memory loss.

Dehydration Can Cause Bad Breath and Other Oral Issues

I certainly didn't expect that drinking more water during my Hydration Challenge would overhaul my oral health, but that's precisely what happened. When you're dehydrated, research shows your body produces less saliva, allowing bacteria and harmful plaque to multiply. This not only causes bad breath but also increases the risk of tooth decay, cavities, gingivitis, and other problems. Not drinking enough can also make it more difficult to swallow food and cause problems for those who wear dentures.

JUNE HYDRATION: Your Story

In theory, this challenge should be relatively easy. After all, we're talking about drinking water here, which requires no physical exertion or mental effort—it's actually something most of us want to do. Another attribute of the month is that water consumption is easy to quantify: you can readily tell if you're meeting your daily hydration if you just keep track of how many glasses or bottles of water you have per day. Still, despite these advantages, proper hydration isn't so straightforward, evidenced by the fact that few of us are meeting our daily water needs. Here are ten ways to start drinking more and make this month even easier than it already is.

1. FIGURE OUT YOUR FORMULA. The IOM recommends women consume 2.7 liters and men 3.7 liters of water daily through food and beverages. But what does that really mean? Since food makes up only 20 percent of our average water intake, most of your daily hydration should come from liquids—and more specifically, from water, which science shows hydrates the body better than beverages that contain sugar, caffeine, artificial sweeteners, or other additives.

    I settled on a daily water target of 2.4 liters for two reasons: (1) I decided that drinking out of water bottles would be the best way for me to quantify that goal, and the bottles I chose were 800 milliliters each, or 2.4 liters total for three, and (2) that total was just slightly below the IOM's recommendation for women, so whatever I ate would more than compensate for the extra 300 milliliters.

What should your daily water target be? I suggest first deciding which vessel you're most likely to drink water out of—glasses, purchased bottles, or refillable water bottles—and then multiply the number of milliliters in the glass or bottle that brings you closest to 2.7 or 3.7 liters, based on your gender. While food will allow you to hover slightly below these recommendations, do not dip below 2.2 liters if you're a woman or 3.2 liters if you're a man. Finally, if you'd rather use the imperial system, 2.2 liters is approximately nine 8-ounce cups, while 3.2 liters is approximately thirteen 8-ounce cups.

2.   DEVELOP A GAME PLAN. Once you set your daily water target, how you meet that goal is entirely up to you. But I recommend devising a game plan before you start. Before the month began, I looked at all aspects of my daily routine and discovered my days were divided into three different segments during which I could consume water: mornings at *GMA*, afternoons in my medical office, and nights at home. From there, it was easy to create a three-bottle strategy, with the goal of finishing one bottle during each segment.

   You might find it easier, however, to find two 8-ounce glasses and keep one at home and the other in the office, drinking a full glass every hour. You can even set a timer on your phone to remind you. Or you may want to carry one water bottle with you everywhere you go, filling it at home, in the office, and out on the road while keeping track of how many refills you finish (see number eight for more advice on how to do this). Or you might prefer to track your water intake with an app like Daily Water Tracker Reminder, Hydro Coach, or Gulp. Most of these apps require you to enter the size or quantity of what you drink and eat and will remind you when you're short on hydration. There are even apps like H2O Pal Water Bottle that pair with "smart" bottles to track how much you drink without any effort on your end.

3.   FIND YOUR PERSONAL WATER PREFERENCE. Before the month began, I used to think water was water was water and that it all pretty much tasted the same. But as it turns out, water is like wine, with many different tastes and varietals, and taking the time to find your preference can make this month easier and more enjoyable—and more sustainable into the future. So experiment with different temperatures— ice cold, cold, lukewarm, and even warm—and different types, whether from the tap, filtered, sparkling, or bottled. You can also try flavoring water with lemon, lime, grapefruit, cucumber, mint, and other fruits, vegetables, or herbs. You can find creative water recipes online with everything from strawberries, ginger, and rose petals to tomato, fennel, and lavender.

4.   DRINK WATER WITH EVERY MEAL. Whether you bring your water bottle to the dinner table or always have a glass with lunch at the office, be sure to drink water at every meal. This is not only an easy and automatic way to boost your intake for the day, it also ensures proper digestion and will slow down the pace at which you eat, increasing feelings of fullness, satiety, and satisfaction.

5.   START PAYING ATTENTION TO YOUR PEE. Don't be afraid to peer at your pee in the toilet—it's one of the best ways to access your overall health. If you're hydrated and healthy, your pee should look pale and straw-colored, similar in hue to a sweat stain on a white T-shirt. If it's darker or a deep yellow, brown, or even maroon color, you're not drinking enough water. If you're consistently meeting the IOM's recommendation yet your urine is still dark, you may be suffering from a medical condition affecting your liver, kidneys, or bladder and should make an appointment with your doctor immediately.

6.   DON'T WORRY ABOUT HAVING TO USE THE BATHROOM. When I started this challenge, I was pleasantly surprised to find out I didn't have to run to the bathroom every hour. While I admittedly had to urinate slightly more than normal, it wasn't an inconvenience, and I rarely woke up more than once a night to use the bathroom—considered healthy for a hydrated person. Living inside a bathroom is a bit of a myth when it comes to hydration—your body has an amazing way of regulating.

7.   INVEST IN A FILTER. You don't need to spend money on bottled water or a water-delivery system to drink more. If you're concerned about tap water or don't like the taste, invest in a filter, which can give hard or mineral-like water the same taste as the bottled stuff from the supermarket. Better still, when you filter water, you avoid drinking water that has sat too long in a plastic bottle or container, reducing your exposure to toxins found in plastic. Do some research to find a filter that best fits your sink and budget, and remember to change the filter regularly, or per manufacturer recommendations. Otherwise, toxins can build up in the filter and eventually overflow into your water.

8.   CUSTOMIZE YOUR WATER BOTTLE TO SEE FIRSTHAND HOW MUCH YOU NEED TO DRINK. If you decide to carry a water bottle with you everywhere you go, you may find it easier to physically mark your hourly time goals on the side of the bottle. Write on tape or use a label maker to print out time goals, then affix them to different levels of the bottle. For example, if you wake up at 8 A.M., affix a label that says 10 A.M. at the sixteen-ounce level of the bottle and aim to drink to that line by that time. You can also now buy water bottles like the Drink More Water Bottle from Uncommon Goods that already include graphics and goals.

9.   DRINK WHILE YOU BREW. I've learned throughout the year
     that a lot can be accomplished while waiting for a cup of
     coffee to brew or the water in your morning shower to turn
     warm. Either way, try to incorporate drinking a full cup of
     water into your morning routine so that you immediately
     start to replenish the water lost during the overnight hours.
     Pairing it with something you do every morning, like mak-
     ing coffee, showering, or putting on makeup, ensures you
     won't forget and will help make the habit as intrinsic to your
     routine as these other activities.

10. CONTINUALLY REMIND YOURSELF HOW MUCH SIPPING IS
     BENEFITING YOUR BODY, BRAIN, HEART, AND SKIN. Drinking
     more water is a tiny investment for gigantic health benefits.
     If you feel yourself flagging in your water intake, remind
     yourself how much hydrating is doing to your body by fuel-
     ing your brain, opening up your veins and heart, flushing
     out your kidneys, softening your skin, priming your mus-
     cles, filling up your stomach, revving your metabolism, and
     keeping every other organ and physical function in your
     body running at optimal levels.

7

More Steps

My Story

Peole who live in New York City do more walking than anyone else in the country, with an average of eight thousand steps per day. In comparison, most Americans take only forty-seven hundred steps daily, according to recent research.

I live in New York City and also work as a health professional, both of which mean I should probably be logging at least eight thousand steps per day. But unfortunately, nothing could be further from the truth.

While I'd never consistently tracked my steps until the More Steps Challenge, whenever I've randomly calculated how much I've walked for the day or week, the number has been pathetically low. In fact, forty-seven hundred steps—average for most Americans—would be a banner day for me. Instead, I seem to hover around three thousand steps daily, even sinking to two thousand on days when I'm slammed with *GMA* and work, forced to take cars instead of walk or use public transport like most New Yorkers do. Also, when I work out, I usually bike or weight train, which doesn't add anything to my daily step count.

For these reasons, trying to take more steps seemed like low-hanging fruit on the challenge tree—something I had to do and from which I knew many others would benefit, too. I also had a month full of travel and long trips, which meant I wouldn't have the chance to get to the gym as often as I'd like. While I had never considered walking a workout, I figured it would help me retain some fitness and burn calories to boot.

I also had a sneakier reason for wanting to walk more. Before the month began, I was heavier on the scale than I'd ever been, except for when I'd been pregnant. I had gained weight on a recent vacation, and I didn't like how it made me look or feel. We weren't talking about a massive amount—only four pounds—but it still bothered me. Also, as a woman in my forties, weight gain could be a slippery slope, when a few extra pounds here suddenly turns into ten or even twenty pounds heavier than you should be. I wanted to nip it in the bud now, and walking seemed like a great supplement to regular exercise and a healthy diet.

While I didn't think it would be physically difficult, I knew a More Steps Challenge would be strenuous from a scheduling standpoint. Typically, my days start with an early-morning ride to *GMA*; I can't walk—the producers won't take a chance with a con-tributor falling into a pothole or getting mugged at the last minute. While I can walk home, it takes about thirty minutes, which is time I rarely have since I start seeing patients at 10 A.M. in my medical office in New Jersey. I also take a car there, as well as home again—unfortunately, you can't walk or take public transport from the city there. Once in my medical office, I walk only twenty or so feet at a time, just to get between exam rooms. I don't have a dedicated lunch break or time for a stroll outside. After I wrap up with work, it's home again and off to SoulCycle or the gym, oftentimes in a car again before I have to rush out for a work or social dinner.

Still, there are times during the week when I can walk. If I don't have patients, I have more time and can walk to afternoon meetings at ABC, which is about thirteen blocks, or fifteen minutes. I can also walk after work if I don't have a dinner or an event to attend, and to SoulCycle on the weekends. But I'll admit, these jaunts are rarities, not regular occurrences.

When thinking about how many steps to set as a daily goal for the month, I wanted a number that would work with my schedule—not so ambitious that I would set myself up for disappointment or failure. The month before I began the challenge, I had averaged five thousand steps daily, with many twenty-five-hundred-step days during the workweek, so shooting for seventy-five hundred steps daily seemed like a reasonable target, given my workload and the fact I already exercised regularly, which alleviated some of the importance of taking ten thousand steps daily. I figured I would keep my iPhone, with its built-in pedometer app, on me at all times, so tracking my progress would be easy.

I was more excited for this challenge than I had been before accomplishing previous ones, primarily because I was motivated to lose a little weight and curious to see if doing something as simple as adding steps would get me there. As a doctor, I was also looking forward to using real-time data to track my progress—with the step counter, I'd know right away whether I was hitting my goal, without room for personal interpretation or opinion. At the same time, though, such lack of subjectivity made me nervous: if I failed, I'd know it, with hard data stored on my iPhone to always remind me.

Week 1
Taking More Steps Is So Much Easier Than You Think

Armed with my step counter and an overwhelming desire to walk off the extra weight, I kicked off the month by logging a lame 4,270 steps. While disappointed, I was not surprised: I had spent the entire day at work, seeing patients, and didn't have time for any extra walking when I got home after a fifteen-hour day. At the same time, 4,270 was better than 2,500, so I knew trying to take more steps—getting up to speak with my nurse, Ana, instead of emailing her and walking Mason a little longer—was at least paying off.

The following day was another long one in the office, but this time, I was determined not to repeat the same results. When I checked my step counter on my drive home and realized I was still painfully below my goal, I hopped on the treadmill in the gym in my building for twenty minutes, which boosted my day's tally to 8,995 steps. Yes! That treadmill was going to become my secret weapon in my war to walk more.

I employed a similar tactic on the third day, walking to SoulCycle and back after seeing I was low on steps after another day in the office, logging a total of 9,457 steps. The next morning, I flew to Canada, but preempted the seven hours I'd spend in the air with endless pacing around the gate, staring at my iPhone nearly the entire time as I watched my step counter climb to 9,366 steps total.

Once in Vancouver, I did something I'd never knowingly done before—I logged 15,360 steps in one day. In the morning, I hit the treadmill at the hotel gym simply because I was unsure how much walking we'd actually do. But once out and about in the city, I decided that my travel companion and I should explore Vancouver on foot. We purposely didn't hail a single cab, and it became a hilarious social challenge as my friend began logging his steps on his phone. When I saw I had netted more than fifteen thousand steps at the end of the day, I was thrilled. Better still, I knew I had experienced and enjoyed more of the city than I ever would have if we'd seen most of it from cabs and cars.

The next day, we walked—or climbed, really—1.8 miles up an infamously grueling Vancouver trail, the Grouse Grind. Given how much I had been sweating and breathing at the summit, I figured I would have logged more than the 8,979 steps for the day, but I wasn't complaining. The last day of the week, I did more than 8,000 steps, but at a much easier clip, circling the Vancouver departure gate before boarding a flight back to New York. Thankfully, I was drinking more water after the June Hydration Challenge—otherwise, all the walking, working out, and traveling likely would have left me with another kidney stone.

When the week was over, I had averaged 8,939 steps per day—a huge improvement over where I'd been the week before, at a paltry average of only 3,854 steps. Moreover, I couldn't believe how easy it had been, despite my slow start and two full travel days. I didn't feel any worse for the wear—no blisters, aches, or pains—and, more important, I felt noticeably more positive, even happier. All that walking and less sitting had increased the blood flow, endorphins, and mood-boosting mitochondrial activity in my brain. Best of all, I had even lost a pound, which was entirely due to taking more steps, as I hadn't made any other changes to my diet or exercise routine.

Week 2
Double Your Steps to Drop Fat and Lose Weight

Bolstered by Week 1's success, I returned to my medical office ready to start Week 2 on a new foot, literally. I checked my counter throughout the day at work, trying to walk even just a few extra steps between exam rooms. When I realized I was still low, I did twenty minutes on the treadmill once I got home. Afterward, I took Mason out for a longer walk, tallying a total of 8,320 steps—more than I'd been able to manage on a workday in a long time.

The next day, though, I logged only 4,333 steps, seeing patients all day, then rushing off for a flight to London at night. I did manage to do some pacing around the airport before we left, but I knew it'd be a disappointing day—I hadn't had time to walk Mason, let alone get on a treadmill or even go to the gym.

I was in London for work, and my itinerary, at least for the first day, was jam-packed. Although there was a gym in the hotel, I didn't have time for the treadmill, let alone my morning meditation that I was still trying to fit in—I rushed out before breakfast, taking a cab across the city to events where I was scheduled to appear. These events continued into the evening, too, and when I finally was able to sink back into my hotel bed at night, I saw I'd been able to manage only 4,468 steps.

The next day, though, I had no work obligations and started the morning exactly the way I wanted: with some meditation, push-ups and planks, and then a ten-minute walk on the hotel treadmill before lifting weights (I was doing slightly less cardio now than during the month of April given my busy schedule, but aerobic workouts were still on my radar). After my gym session, I set out to see London on foot, taking only two taxis the entire day—and simply because I couldn't walk to meet friends in time. This was a deviation from the norm—my standard is to take cabs everywhere—but opting to be bipedal produced big results, as I tracked 13,181 steps that day.

Then it was back to work, as I hailed a cab first thing the following morning to an all-day event on the other side of the city. In the taxicab back to the hotel after dinner, I checked my step counter, and the number was so pathetically low that, despite how late it was, I decided I had to drag myself to the gym treadmill for a thirty-minute walk. Even with this longer jaunt, I went to bed with only 3,634 steps. At this point, the battle in walking warfare was obvious: it was work versus steps. And since work wasn't optional, I had to figure out how to get more steps on even my busiest days.

Thankfully, the next day included only a few hours of work in the afternoon for a *GMA* appearance. That morning, I decided to walk from my hotel to the Tower of London. The castle, if you've never been, is immense, and the only way to see it is on foot, so we spent several hours walking around the grounds and seeing everything inside the fortress, palace, and prison. After the *GMA* taping, we went to lunch in Notting Hill. I had been to that area of London before, but it was such a pleasant day—and I was, after all, still a tourist—that I suggested walking around afterward to window-shop. As we did so, I thought to myself how easy and enjoyable it would be to do this at home with family or friends, even in those neighborhoods I already knew. At the end of the day, I had 17,450 steps for the day—a new record for the month.

Finally, it was time to fly home. We landed in New York in the morning, and despite my jet lag, I squeezed in a walk to SoulCycle (cardio session!) and back to my apartment to end the day at 5,113 steps. This was unusual for me: I had just flown across a major ocean after spending days in three different time zones across the world, yet I was still full of energy. My only explanation was the walking, even though I was continuing to drink more water. I felt revitalized, even though I'd spent thirty hours cumulatively on a plane since the challenge began.

After I got back from London, I weighed myself: I had lost another pound and a half. This was more impressive than the energy boost, or that I'd managed to drop two and a half pounds in two weeks simply by walking more. I wasn't able to go to the gym as often I wanted with the insane travel schedule and I certainly wasn't restricting my diet since I had been eating out nearly every night and at events—and I hadn't dropped my monthly intent from May to choose healthier plant foods over red meat when possible.

I did, however, end the week with a big blister on one foot, which was entirely my fault: in London I had worn sneakers strictly meant for fashion, not fitness. More so, I was frustrated I still hadn't been able to log more steps during busy days, but I had learned a good lesson— that it was possible to make up steps on the days I had off, like I did in London. And while I had logged my biggest step days while sightseeing, I felt confident I could adapt certain activities, like taking a postmeal stroll, in New York.

Week 3
How More Steps Can Suppress Appetite and Kill Cravings

The week started with consecutive mornings on *GMA*, then long hours in my medical office both days as I saw patients I'd been unable to see the previous week. My steps were consistent with busy workdays, as I tallied only 3,889 steps the first day and 4,963 steps the second.

Midway through the week, I took another night flight, this time to Paris, fitting in a quick twenty-minute walk on the treadmill before I had to head to the airport. I tried to add some extra steps while waiting to board, but when I took my seat, I had only 4,584 steps for the day. I was disappointed the week now seemed to be off to a bumpy start, but I knew, as I tried to get some sleep on the plane, that I would be able to walk as much as I wanted in Paris. The trip was purely for pleasure—a short vacation with my friend Laura—and it would be great to see the city in a way I never had before.

If there was a theme to the next three days, it would have been *Vive le Marche:* all we did was walk. Laura was generous enough to allow me to lead her just about everywhere on two feet, which we did to nearly all our destinations. She had a Fitbit, so we spent many hours over *café* comparing how many steps her device reported she took compared to my iPhone. Interestingly, the step counter was consistently 20–25 percent lower in steps than the Fitbit, which made me feel better about my pathetic walking days earlier in the week. And it made me even more impressed by what we did in Paris, logging 16,513 steps the first day, 10,401 steps the second day, and 19,021 steps on the last day—my record for the month to date.

On the plane home, I was definitely fatigued from all the walking, but I didn't have any aches or pains, not even in my knees. I also didn't have a single blister: I had worn gym sneakers almost the entire time, purposely planning my outfits so I wouldn't look like a tacky American tourist but wouldn't feel hindered when I walked. That last day, I logged only 3,412 steps, but I wasn't upset. Instead, I looked at my weekly average, which was an impressive, for me, 9,212 steps.

After Paris, I also felt my appetite drop. It was already low after my June hydration month, but this was getting impressive: despite spending three days in a country known for its butter croissants, chocolate soufflés, and other rich food, I hadn't been as tempted by these treats as I normally would have been. Plus, I was far more mindful about my wine consumption, after January's dry month, so I wasn't consuming as many calories from alcohol as I might normally while on vacation.

At the end of the week, I had lost another pound and a half—while taking a trip to Paris, of all times. I felt physically lighter on my feet while my energy levels continued to increase. My success so far was also mentally gratifying, partly because I had lost weight, but also because I knew, without a doubt, that I was getting this challenge, thanks to the step counter.

Week 4
How Walking More Can Create Happiness

The last week started the same as the majority of the month: on a plane. I had to be in Los Angeles for work, so after getting home from Paris the day before, I hopped an early-morning flight to L.A. the next day, getting in some steps at the airport for 4,229 total steps.

The good thing about the trip, while for work, was that it primarily took place at the University of California, Los Angeles, and the only way to get from one event to the next was on foot. For extra assurance, I still did a thirty-minute walk on the hotel treadmill in the morning, but it wasn't necessary, as it turned out. I was already above my daily goal by midday, but I still suggested walking 1.6 miles from campus to a local restaurant where I was taking my staff to dinner. While my default would have been to a taxi, I now wanted to walk whenever I had the time, an attitude that helped me end the day with 9,620 steps.

The following day started ridiculously early—with a 3:30 A.M.

alarm for an early-morning flight back to New York—and any treadmill time, let alone meditation or any other healthy morning habits, was out of the question. After landing in the city, I jumped in a cab home, quickly changed clothes, then hailed another taxi downtown, only to arrive slightly late to a charity event I was emceeing. The day was the worst for the month so far—only 2,771 steps—but I decided not to let it bother me. Mentally, I knew I was already doing well for the month and I was learning you just can't get blood from a stone on a schedule-crazy day.

The next day, I saw patients for hours on end, but managed a few walks with Mason for 5,803 steps total. Then it was back to the airport the following morning to hop a flight to Detroit, where Chloe had hockey games all weekend. I had much more time in the terminal than I had before the L.A. flight, so I paced around the gate before taking off, then landing in Detroit. The Detroit terminal, if you've ever been, is extensive, so I logged several hundred steps just trying to get from Arrivals to the rental-car counter. Then, Chloe always has to be at the rink exceedingly early, so I paced around waiting for her game to begin, switching seats every quarter once it did, adding more steps. At the end of the day, despite the travel, I was only four hundred steps below my goal: 7,099.

The first full day in Detroit, I logged 9,073 steps by hitting the treadmill for thirty minutes, then walking around the rink and the city for meals. The next day, Chloe had a game in the morning, so I did some more rink pacing, then we walked to brunch at the renowned Hudson Cafe. Next it was off to the airport, but we got there so early that I left my bags with Chloe and walked the length of that extensive Detroit terminal . . . twice. I was already over my 7,500 steps, but I wanted to (1) kill time and (2) burn extra calories since I wouldn't get to the gym that day. When I passed another hockey parent who was also a fitness buff, we shared a communal chuckle because he knew exactly what I was doing: with athletic daughters on a demanding sports team, our fitness routines had been relegated to walking airport workouts. But I didn't mind, especially when I saw I'd logged 9,689 steps that day.

The next two days, I tallied 8,907 and 8,806 steps with more walking on the treadmill and trying to take extra steps at work. Then, on the very last day of the month, when I realized I was below 7,500, I took Mason up onto the rooftop of my apartment building at night, high up over all the sparkling lights of New York City, and walked him around the perimeter until I was sure I'd hit 7,523 steps.

At the end of the month, I had averaged 8,284 steps a day for the entire period. I felt more positive and upbeat than I could remember in a long time and proud that I'd done something I'd never considered a health-and-wellness priority. Sure, I knew walking was important to basic health, but I considered it to be like eating or breathing—an activity you need to do to live rather than to stay active or even improve your fitness and health. I had never imagined taking more steps would impart the benefits it did and even take the place of a traditional workout on those days when I was too time-strapped to get to the gym.

What four weeks of consistent walking had done for me, in short, was overhaul how I looked and felt. I've always been an energetic person, but when I started moving more and sitting less, the extra activity boosted my energy levels by at least 25 percent. At the same time, I felt calmer, like walking was a type of movement meditation.

I'd also lost two and a half pounds—impressive in a month when I'd traveled extensively, including several pleasure trips, and not been able to work out as much. My stomach felt flatter, too, and the only thing I had done differently was walk more. Yet despite all the walking, I didn't have any aches or pains other than my one London blister, which receded after I began paying attention to my footwear. Perhaps most important, I loved walking more throughout life. It made me happier, and I no longer felt like the month's challenge was a chore or something I had to discipline myself to do.

JULY MORE STEPS:
The Science Behind Taking More Steps

I n the last decade, multiple studies have shown how Americans don't walk enough and how this inactivity is taking a toll on our collective health. Headlines like "Sitting Is as Bad as Smoking," "15 Minutes of Walking a Day Could Save Your Life," and "Sitting Is the New Cancer," while hyperbolic, have called attention to the fact we're sitting way too much and not walking as much as we need to to stay healthy and prevent weight gain and chronic disease like cancer, Alzheimer's, and heart disease. Yet there are other more surprising benefits to walking more. All you need is two feet—no special equipment or gym membership—to lose weight and get on a path, literally, to better health.

Walking Can Help You Lose More Weight Than You Think

Much of recent hubbub around weight loss has centered on low-carb eating and high-intensity intervals—two approaches that require significant discipline and lifestyle modifications and are massively incomplete when it comes to solving the complex disorders of being overweight or obese. While both have plenty of scientific merit, weight management experts also know that the tried and true, like simply moving more, can also have big benefits for your waistline.

For example, a 2002 study from researchers at the University of Miami found that people who walked at a moderate pace for only three hours a week—the equivalent of approximately 18,000–27,000 steps per week, or 2,600–3,900 steps per day—lost significantly more weight than those who consumed the same number of calories but didn't add more steps. Those who walked also had lower levels of cholesterol and insulin, the body's fat-storing hormone, at the end of the three-month study.

How can walking help you lose weight? Quite simply, it helps your body burn more calories. According to the American Council on

Exercise (ACE), a 140-pound person burns 7.6 calories per minute when walking at a pace of 13:20 minutes per mile, or 228 calories for a thirty-minute walk. Experts at ACE also say you can burn up to 3,500 calories per week—the equivalent of one pound of pure fat loss—simply by logging 10,000 steps per day.

Walking may even help you lose weight on a cellular level. Researchers at Harvard University discovered that people who walked briskly for an hour a day cut the effects of over thirty obesity-promoting genes in half—in other words, walking helped outsmart a genetic predisposition to obesity. Don't have an hour to walk? Don't worry. The Harvard study also found obesity genes were most active in those who walked the least, meaning that more steps, no matter how many, only lessens the impact of weight-gaining DNA.

Take More Steps to Cut Cravings, Slow Hunger, and Curb Weight Gain

Despite the misconception otherwise, exercise is one of the most effective ways to suppress appetite, helping slash hunger not only following a workout but for hours afterward, too. Better still, you don't have to break a sweat to get exercise's appetite-abating effects: research shows that walking is a particularly effective way to quell cravings and hunger. A 2012 study out of Brigham Young University found that when people walked in the morning, their brains responded less to images of tasty food than on the days they didn't walk. Another 2015 study from researchers at the University of Innsbruck in Austria discovered that walking briskly for only fifteen minutes can cut cravings for sugary snacks.

Walking Reduces Breast Cancer Risk

You may already know that exercise is a great preventive measure against breast cancer. But a recent study found that walking in particular can also cut breast cancer occurrence, even in the most vulnerable populations. Researchers found that postmenopausal women who walked at least seven hours a week had a 14 percent lower chance of developing breast cancer than their more sedentary counterparts. Another study of approximately eighty thousand walkers and runners found that those who met the CDC guidelines for exercise—which recommend Americans exercise moderately for two and a half hours or vigorously for an hour and fifteen minutes per week—were 42 percent less likely to die of breast cancer over an eleven-year period than those who didn't meet the CDC standards.

Walking Boosts Your Mood, No Matter Where or When You Do It

As I discovered, walking can have a profound effect on how you feel and look at the world—and it doesn't matter how down in the dumps you are or whether you walk only around your equally dreary office. A 2016 study published in the journal *Emotion* found that walking boosts positive affect—how much we're able to experience positivity—making us feel more energized, engaged, enthusiastic, and open to joy, regardless of current mood or the environment in which we walk. Researchers concluded that even a quick walk around drab office halls or gray suburban streets can be uplifting and produce feelings of happiness.

Walking doesn't just make you happy—it can also help fight depression, anxiety, and stress. According to the Anxiety and Depression Association of America, researchers have found that taking a ten-minute walk can reduce feelings of depression, fatigue, and anger and suppress anxiety as effectively as a forty-five-minute workout. The effects of a short, brisk walk don't just go away once we get back to the office or our homes—scientists say the effects of walking on mood can last for hours after a single jaunt.

Walking Can Make You Smarter

One reason I enjoyed walking during the More Steps Challenge is that it helped me think more clearly. Turns out, taking more steps can help improve cognitive performance, researchers say, in part by increasing the flow of blood, oxygen, and nutrients to the brain. Regular walking also triggers the growth of new neurons and connections between brain cells while increasing the size of your brain's hippocampus (which controls memory) and preventing age-related tissue decline. For these reasons, researchers have found that walking can help boost mental alertness and memory.

Struggling to come up with a solution or a new strategy? Try taking a walk. In 2014 researchers at Stanford University found that walking can increase creative output by up to an average of 60 percent. The scientists concluded that it was the act of walking, not necessarily the scenery, that triggered more expansive thinking, since participants were walking on treadmills.

Walking Boosts Bone Density in Ways Other Exercise Does Not

I have lots of patients who are very active, always cycling, swimming, or rowing out on the Hudson River. And while I commend them for the exercise, I also remind them that these activities won't improve their bone health because they're not weight-bearing. That's where walking comes in. Walking, like running, weight lifting, dancing, and other impact activities, stresses bones, which stimulates cells to grow, thereby building bone strength. But you don't have to jump or sprint to get the benefits. One 1994 study published in *The American Journal of Medicine* found that women who walked just a mile a day had better whole-body bone density than those who walked shorter distances. A 2002 study from researchers at Brigham and Women's Hospital found that walking reduces the risk of hip fractures by 30 percent. For my patients with osteopenia or osteoporosis, I recommend wearing a weighted vest when they walk or even grocery shop to add more positive weight-bearing stress on their bones.

JULY MORE STEPS: Your Story

How Many Steps Should You Take Per Day?

While ten thousand steps per day may be the most commonly prescribed number for good health, if you don't currently walk much now, that goal may be too ambitious. Before you begin this month's challenge, track your current number of steps by using the free pedometer app on your smartphone or investing in a wearable tracking device (see tip number one below). If you're taking fewer than two thousand steps per day, start with a daily target of thirty-five hundred and increase by five hundred steps per week until you hit five thousand—the minimum experts say we need to be fit and healthier.

Walking is so simple to do—and so simple to fit into your life if you just start prioritizing it. Think about it this way: even if your lifestyle doesn't include a lot of walking now, the only way to get from point A to point B, even if it's just from your bedroom to the car, is by walking. That means you can get more steps just by walking slightly farther in every walk you take. Yet since that's often easier said than done, here are ten ways to work more walking into your everyday life.

1. FIND A TRACKING DEVICE THAT WORKS FOR YOU. The free step counter on my phone was a lifesaver for the More Steps Challenge, allowing me to quickly and easily track my steps every day. Having hard evidence of how many steps I'd

taken toward my daily goal motivated me to walk more and gave me a gratifying sense of success whenever I went over seventy-five hundred. Nearly all iPhones have a built-in pedometer—find it under the Health application—or there are countless free step apps you can download to your smartphone. If you'd rather go phone-free, consider investing in a wearable tracking device like a Fitbit or Apple watch.

2. LOOK AT EVERY CHORE, DAILY ROUTINE, AND PHONE CALL AS POSSIBLE STEP TIME. You've heard the suggestions before: park your car far away from the office or store, opt for the stairs over the elevator, and walk to see a colleague instead of emailing. It's time-old advice, but it's time-old for a reason: it works. Adding more steps to your daily chores and routines is the easiest, most seamless way to walk more. Look at errands or household chores as fun opportunities to rack up the count on your pedometer or Fitbit. For example, how many steps can you get during a trip to the bank or while putting away the family's laundry? Finally, use all your phone calls, whether personal or at work, to walk and talk, whether around your home or the office.

3. WALK YOUR DOG—FOR REAL. Before I started this challenge, I mostly took Mason out just to pee or poop, which, other than preventing messes, didn't really benefit the dog—or me. But I've now started walking him, which only takes me five more minutes, to give him the walk we both desperately need. This month, instead of ambling about while waiting for Spot or Daisy to do his or her thing, use the time to really walk your pup, taking a few more minutes than you normally do. After all, you're already outside and walking, and five more minutes wouldn't break your schedule—but will give you five hundred more steps.

4. RETHINK YOUR FOOTWEAR. I realized pretty quickly that I couldn't go for a spontaneous, long walk if I was wearing work heels or sneakers designed for fashion, not fitness. That's why I started carrying gym shoes with me everywhere—to the office, across town to meet friends, whenever I traveled—or wearing gym shoes and slipping on heels I carried in my purse before meeting friends or colleagues. While you may think you can walk five thousand, seven thousand, or even ten thousand steps a day in ballet flats or cute biker boots, if you do it day after day for the entire month, your feet—and your joints, bones, and muscles—may convince you otherwise.

5. PAD IN TIME TO WALK THERE. While it takes only twenty minutes to walk one mile, most of us don't do it whenever we have to run out to the store, want coffee, or go to the gym. The reason for our laziness is often convenience rather than lack of time—after all, the average American spends hours every day watching TV and scrolling through social media. But if you don't build in the time to walk, it won't happen. I found I was more successful in racking up steps on the days I strategically built in twenty more minutes to a daily activity, like a SoulCycle class or a meeting at ABC, so I could walk there instead of taking a car or a cab.

6. TURN YOUR CHALLENGE INTO SOMETHING SOCIAL FOR MORE STEPS. When I told my family, friends, and colleagues I was doing the challenge, the response was great—many were eager to join, whether for just a two-hour lunch or a full three-day trip. This was a fantastic source of support and also turned the challenge into a fun team effort. While in Paris with Laura, we had a blast checking our steps throughout the day, comparing her Fitbit to my iPhone and celebrating whenever we tracked lots of walking. Back home, friends and I would take pre- or postdinner walks, which turned

out to give us more quality time than we would have had sharing a cab or even having a second drink. There are other ways I could have socialized the challenge, too. For example, if you routinely meet a friend or colleague for coffee, try taking your beverage for a walk. Or in lieu of meeting at a friend's home for lunch, suggest a walk-and-talk to a picnic at a local park. The options are endless if you start thinking steps first.

7. TAKE IT ONE DAY AT A TIME BUT KEEP THE BIG PICTURE IN VIEW. The only thing you can do is try to walk as much as you can every single day this month. But there will likely be some days when you won't be able to meet your goal—you're sick, the weather is horrible, or you're just too slammed with life to take the steps you want. Don't get discouraged or beat yourself up about it. I found it easy to make up for lost steps on the weekends or when I had quiet days. There are thirty-one days in July, so if you have one bad day, remember you have a few dozen more to try to get in the walking you want to do.

8. TURN WAITING INTO WALKING. Everyone spends a portion of every day waiting for something or someone, whether it's for a colleague, family member, or friend, a coffee, a flight, an elevator, in your car for your kids . . . The list goes on. I learned that turning these idle times into walking waits is an easy way to rack up more steps. Better still, I truly enjoyed the wait more when I spent it pacing around the Vancouver, London, and Detroit airports.

9. FIND YOUR SECRET WALKING WEAPON. My secret weapon this month was the treadmill in my apartment building. Whenever I was low in steps, hitting the treadmill for twenty to thirty minutes was a fast, easy, and simple way to rack up

several thousand steps at one time. While I know not everyone has easy access to a treadmill, it's not the only way to bank a big chunk of steps at one time. Lisa Lillien, author of the *Hungry Girl* blog, has popularized housewalking—simply walking around your home—as an easy way to rack up steps. Others like to use running tracks, indoor or outdoor shopping malls, or local parks to build steps.

10. STEP SAFELY. Walking is critical to good health, but not if or when it puts your life or limbs in jeopardy. That's why I recommend never walking in unfamiliar neighborhoods at night or alone. Also, no matter where you live, you shouldn't walk and text. After this month's challenge, I made a rule with my kids that we would never walk and text—there are just too many potential dangers, including speeding cars, bicycles, potholes, construction sites, and sudden intersections. Even if you don't live in an urban area, walking while buried in your phone will distract you from your surroundings, which could include threats like angry dogs, swerving cars, or people who might not have your best interest at heart.

8

Mindful Tech

My Story

During my last few years at ABC, I've been surrounded by the news and, consequently, lots of talk about America's collective addiction to technology. In short, we're always on our phones, laptops, desktops, iPads, Apple watches, and other devices, oftentimes for no good reason, and it's killing our mental, physical, emotional, and social health. My kids call it *phubbing*, or snubbing others in social situations because you're too busy on your phone. (Note: This term is not just one coined by Gen Z but is widely used in media and even in some medical articles on technology addiction.) And unfortunately, the word comes up with my kids because, unlike most parent-child interactions, I'm usually the one buried in my phone, causing my kids to get annoyed and offended. And they are right to feel that way!

While it's no excuse, the reason I'm often attached to my phone is that, as a doctor, my patients' health needs don't always adhere to a nine-to-five, Monday-through-Friday schedule. I also have a separate work phone for ABC, where I have to be on call 24/7 for last-minute medical questions, breaking medical news, and segment appearances. To perform well at both of my jobs, I need constantly to be connected to two phones. Going off the grid entirely isn't an option for me. Ever.

But when I began to think about my day-to-day tech consumption, I knew I had a problem. On any given day, I receive hundreds of emails, 99 percent of which require a response. Not every email necessitates an immediate reply, but sometimes it's difficult to tell which ones are urgent and which can be answered later in the day or even week. I also receive up to twenty different texts per day, many that require some back-and-forth. Like just about everyone who owns a mobile device, I also use my cell phone for social media, 70 percent of which is for work and about 30 percent is personal. I try to respond to my followers on Twitter and Instagram when I can, and I also like to check Twitter once every few hours to stay current on the latest medical news. I also have two Facebook pages, one for professional use and one for personal. Finally, I use my phone like a laptop, looking up the day's news and researching medical topics for a friend or patient or before a *GMA* segment.

I even keep my phone by my bed at night and check it as soon as I wake up. I stay on my phone while I'm getting ready, in the car to *GMA*, even in the elevator up to the studio. I work on my phone through lunch in my medical office, sometimes even using my desktop computer and phone at the same time. I never seem to be able to walk to work or the gym without texting, reading, or emailing, and when I get home, the phone is with me at the dinner table and even when I climb into bed. In short, if I'm not on-air for *GMA* or speaking with a patient in my office, most of the time, I'm on my phone.

The worst of it was that I knew my phone was interfering with my personal relationships and preventing me from enjoying the moment, noticing my surroundings, and fully appreciating my food, family, and friends. I became more aware of my habits not only because I constantly got busted by my own teenage kid, but also after spending time with my boyfriend. With him, my phone seemed to disappear—I would go hours without looking at it. This meant, shockingly, that I was actually living in the moment. How refreshing! On some level, I suspected my phone use was also affecting my health. That, I decided, made learning to use my phone more mindfully the perfect challenge.

The difficult part, though, was devising an actual challenge that would allow me to rely on my phone less. Consuming less technology is an immensely personal pursuit: we all have different professional and personal demands that mandate when and where we need our phones, laptops, tablets, computers, and other gizmos and gadgets. Personally, I knew I couldn't unplug entirely, so to create a goal for this month, I had to examine closely my schedule and lifestyle to figure out when it made the most sense for me, Jen, to go without my phone.

For me, the most obvious time I didn't need to be on my phone was whenever I was walking through New York City—something I was trying to do much more often after my More Steps Challenge. From all the walking I had done last month, I had learned that staring at my phone while doing so wasn't just a hazard—more than five thousand people have been killed and eleven thousand injured while walking and texting in the last decade—it was also unnecessary. Was I really going to miss something dire in the fifteen minutes it took to stroll up to a SoulCycle class or to walk to my ABC office? And if I did receive an email or text I had to respond to, could I really devise an apt answer while trying to get where I was going on time and avoiding cabs, cars, potholes, and other pedestrians at the same time? Absolutely not.

But similar to May's Less Meat, More Plants Challenge, I didn't want to just eliminate something—my phone, in this instance—without adding something positive in its place. While I vowed to walk phone-free for the month, I resolved to do so by focusing on enjoying my surroundings more when I walked—something I realized I hadn't done in years. New York in August is warm and bustling, and you never know what or whom you'll see: a celebrity sighting, a new restaurant, a beautiful sunset over the Hudson. But you have to be paying attention. I wasn't even appreciating some of the city's most iconic landmarks. For example, how many times had I walked by the stunning campus of Lincoln Center without even really looking at it?

I figured I'd start with this target—to avoid using my phone whenever I walked—and then I could evolve the challenge as the month progressed and I hopefully discovered new ways to be more present without technology.

Week 1
The Unbelievable Benefits of Going Phone-Free for Just Thirty Minutes

---

The first day of the month was warm and sunny—a perfect morning for a summer walk from my apartment to ABC on the Upper West Side. As I left, though, I had to verbally remind myself to put my phone in my purse. After all, with the amount I was using it, my phone was no longer an accessory but an appendage.

But once my phone was stowed and I was walking, I felt like a tourist in my own city. I had walked the same fifteen minutes to ABC many times and knew the route by rote, but I had never done it without my head buried in my phone. I was immediately struck by the sight of Lincoln Center, which looked like a dazzling ancient temple in the morning light. The streets were just starting to whirl with people, as cafés opened their doors and stocked sidewalks with tables and chairs and food vendors rolled their carts into place to serve coffee and pretzels for the day. It was as if a whole new New York suddenly opened up, one that I'd loved for years, but hadn't truly seen in months.

During that first walk, I didn't pull out my phone once, even though I knew people had texted and emailed. As soon as I got into the elevator at ABC, though, I took out my phone, a little panicky I might have missed something critical. But when I realized nothing earth-shattering had happened in that quarter hour, I was reassured about my potential for success going forward.

Four days that week, I walked to and from ABC or to and from SoulCycle, the latter which was about a thirty-minute walk each way. Once my phone was in my bag, I had no problem keeping it there, but I still had to remind myself every day to put it in my purse, since it was like instant muscle memory to have it in my hand.

For the rest of the week, when I wasn't on my phone-free walks, I allowed myself normal device use. But I tried to be more conscious of phubbing, resisting the urge to pick up my phone whenever it rang, beeped, or dinged during outings with family or friends.

As the week went on, I started to feel calmer during and after my phone-free walks—the commute was peaceful, not stressful as it had been when I was on my phone, trying to answer texts and emails while dodging people, potholes, bike messengers, and moving traffic. This had a cumulative effect, as I was suddenly enjoying thirty minutes to a full hour of serenity most days of the week. The benefits of going without my phone were similar to those I had experienced during my meditation month: I was more relaxed by the end of the week and better able to tackle stress when it did arise. I was also getting to know the city like I never had before, noticing restaurants and shops that had undoubtedly been there for years, but that I'd never seen.

At the end of the week, though, I realized this challenge was different from others to date: I was uncertain how to structure it going forward. I wanted to limit my phone use beyond my around-town walks but didn't know how to do it logistically without jeopardizing my responsibilities to my patients or to ABC. I wasn't daunted by this hurdle, though, but excited to experiment and find a way to be more mindful about my phone.

Week 2

Make Your Bed for Sleeping, Not Stressing Over Your Phone

I couldn't stop thinking about how to make the month's challenge more effective. For example, should I designate certain hours every day to be phone-free? Or should I set a timer and check email only when it beeps, reading and responding at the same time? I spent the first few days of the second week weighing these options while continuing to take my phone-free walks.

By the middle of the week, I had found one solution: there was no need to be on my phone before bed. I knew phones and other screens can disrupt sleep, but I also figured if I hadn't seen an email or Instagram post by the time I was getting into bed, usually around 9 P.M., it could wait until the next day. Also, why did I want to read potentially stressful emails before bed, anyway? I resolved I would still bring my phone into my bedroom, though, on the chance ABC had a question about the next day's segment or my kids needed to reach me.

During this newly acquired free time before bed, I started thinking about why I felt compelled to respond to emails and texts sent late at night or early in the morning. Did the sender really expect a reply at 12:30 A.M. or 4:30 A.M.? Probably not. But then why send a missive at that time? Admittedly, I was guilty of doing the same after I got up at 5 A.M. This month, I decided to be more mindful and considerate of how and when I used my phone.

That week, I completed three round-trip phone-free walks—two to ABC and a third to SoulCycle. The other days, I was too busy at work to get in a walk, and I didn't make it to SoulCycle over the weekend, which obviated a fourth or fifth jaunt. The good news, though, is that it was becoming more automatic to stow my phone in my bag when I did walk, even though it still felt slightly unnatural.

I was still curious to find more ways to address my phone addiction. Ironically—although perhaps not surprisingly—I began to wonder whether some sort of technology existed that would help me reduce my dependency on technology. Truthfully, if I could wear a handheld buzzer that would shock me every time I reached for my phone, I would snatch it up in a second.

Overall, I still liked my strategy—the phone-free walks and no-email nights—because it was sustainable. It meant I was successfully reducing my phone consumption in a way I could continue into the next month while increasing my awareness of, and consequently my concern about, how much I was using my phone the rest of the day. Similar to how my Dry Challenge made me realize how much more alcohol I was drinking per glass, this month was opening my eyes to exactly how much I was using my phone and how it was affecting my relationships and social life.

Week 3
Less Phone Means More Time for Family and Friends

As I continued to reduce how much I used my phone at night, I began to struggle with the idea of what to do with my newfound free time. I now realized I had actually felt productive when I'd been checking my email every two minutes at night, concurrently paging back and forth between all my social media accounts. But I knew this was absurd: What had I been accomplishing other than acting like a crazy phone addict?

But without the diversion of maniacally scrolling through my phone, I felt out of sorts, like I wasn't doing something that I should be. Was this what it meant to be in the moment? And if I am truly in the moment, does that mean I'm being productive? These were the kinds of questions I began to consider during my phone-free nights. I wasn't coming to any answers yet, which I thought was better—I wanted to mull these experiences over—because I knew the conclusions I came to could be potentially life-altering.

I was particularly introspective about my free time during the third week because I didn't have a single business or social dinner, which was a rare occasion. At times, I felt fortunate to have relaxing downtime, but on other nights, I was fidgety and concerned that I didn't have anything to do. I tried to check in with my past challenges, using the time to take extra steps if I was low, to schedule an aerobic workout, or even to meditate or do push-ups and planks at night if I hadn't already in the morning.

At the end of the third week, I went to Cape Cod for a long weekend to visit Chloe, who was there for hockey training camp. Before I left, I wondered if the trip would cause me to feel more panicky about trying to be less connected out of the city, or if, conversely, I would feel more carefree. I hadn't seen Chloe in a while, though, and wanted to be present when I did. I also secretly hoped she'd notice my phubbing and phone habits had improved.

Turns out, I spent less time on my phone and more time with my daughter for the full weekend. I also felt calmer and more engaged in the moment, which wasn't because I was just on vacation—when I'm out of the city, I often feel more frenetic because I'm worried something will go wrong and I'm too far away from my patients or the ABC studios to do anything to help. To me, this meant the challenge was working. Perhaps more to the point, my daughter noticed I was more mindful and in the moment—the best possible gift that could come of any challenge.

Week 4
Go Tech-Free to Transform Leisure Time from Fun to Phenomenal

My excursion to Cape Cod was quickly followed by a nine-day vacation to Italy. I hadn't been on an extended trip that wasn't work-related since college—and I was ecstatic. I was also curious to see how I'd handle my phone. In the past, I had taken shorter vacations to spas and resorts that had a phone-free policy, meaning you couldn't use your device in public spaces, only in your room. Although we weren't going to a phone-free resort, I was traveling with my boyfriend and wanted to be as present as possible, as much for his sake as for my own. And I wanted to end the month by giving the challenge all I could.

Before we left New York, I did something I'd never done before: I set an out-of-office reply for my email, for both work and ABC. Prior to this challenge, I would have never dreamed of cutting myself off from communication, even if I was headed out of the country. But I really wanted to unplug in Italy, even if I was admittedly nervous the world would somehow implode while I was gone. I reminded myself that millions of successful, busy people use out-of-office replies, and their businesses, practices, and political campaigns somehow manage to survive.

Once in Italy, I decided to keep my phone on me (with my step counter active!) and still check for texts in case my kids or parents needed me. But because of the time difference between Europe and the United States—and also because I had told nearly everyone I knew about my mindful tech month—I didn't expect to receive a lot of correspondence.

During the trip, I checked my email only twice, both times more to make sure the out-of-office reply was still working than to see if I had missed anything earth-shattering. I posted a few pictures on Instagram but didn't take the time to scroll through my feed or answer any comments. And I entirely ignored Twitter—I figured if something significant happened in my field or the world at large, I would hear about it in Italy, too.

The end result was amazing: I felt more engaged, in the moment, and relaxed than I had on previous vacations. Although it was a longer vacation than I'd taken in years and I knew absolutely no one was expecting a response or correspondence from me, the reality that the world was still rotating on its axis without my typical technology use was an unbelievable revelation.

I realized something else during the week: despite traveling, schlepping around luggage, and sleeping in new beds, I ended the week feeling looser and more limber than I had in some time, without the chronic stiff neck I seem to suffer from continually looking down at my phone. My posture was straighter, too, because my shoulders weren't humped over as a result of staring down too long at a screen. The increased walking and continued push-ups and planks were inevitably improving my posture, too, but not using my phone as much was straightening out my upper torso and neck in amazing ways.

At the end of the month, I resolved I had to continue to curtail my phone addiction. I was more focused and engaged than I had been in years, able to enjoy what I was doing while I was doing it. While I'd been worried at first whether I was still being productive, by the end of the month I realized I was actually more productive. Taking the time to be alone and really allow myself to think and be creative, instead of spending those minutes mindlessly on my phone, gave me the mental space to consider the issues in my life, come up with solutions, and tackle tasks that make my life better. I may have felt my phone use was making me more productive, but in reality, as I learned this month, it was stealing my time and preventing me from experiencing a more fulfilling, thoughtful life.

The benefits of this challenge were twofold, too. By the end of the month, my friends and especially my children were grateful I was now able to put my phone down and be present when we spent time together. This, in turn, became something I noticed among other people in public, at restaurants, on trains, and out in the streets, when people seemed to have no awareness of others around them because they were so buried in their phones. I used to be one of those people, but now, I told myself, never again.

AUGUST MINDFUL TECH:
The Science Behind More Mindful Tech

The average American spends up to five hours cumulatively on his or her phone every day. According to data compiled by Apple, iPhone users check their devices eighty times per day or three hundred thousand times per year. As far as social media goes, nearly 75 percent of Facebook users visit the site every day, while more than half check multiple times daily. Bottom line: if you think you don't have a problem, you may want to reconsider. And even if you're positive you don't have a problem, reducing your technology consumption by learning more mindful habits still has a multitude of benefits, as science shows.

Yes, You Can Be Addicted to Technology—and the Side Effects Can Be Just as Bad as Drugs

When it comes to addiction, most of us think of drugs, alcohol, cigarettes, gambling, even sex and sugar. We rarely consider technology, even though cell phones, which are owned by 95 percent of Americans, and social media, used by nearly 70 percent of the country, are more prolific than some of these other vices like alcohol, which only 56 percent of us consumed in the last month. According to the Center for Internet and Technology Addiction, 90 percent of all Americans overuse, abuse, or misuse smartphones, computers, social media, and the Internet.

Technology addiction isn't a modern-day theory, but a real condition that can cause serious health effects, including clinical anxiety, depression, insomnia, mood swings, social isolation, loneliness, weight gain or loss, neck or back pain, carpal tunnel syndrome, headaches, vision problems, and an increased risk of suicide.

Your Smartphone May Be Making You Stupid

According to technology expert Nicholas Carr in a 2017 *Wall Street Journal* article, "How Smartphones Hijack Our Minds," our phones have allowed us to rarely flex our memory muscle, as everything we need to know or remember can easily be pulled up on a device. This, he concludes, has led to the reality that "no matter how much information swirls around us, the less well-stocked our memory, the less we have to think with."

Carr isn't the only one to blame smartphones for eroding our intelligence. A 2017 study from researchers at the University of Texas at Austin found that people's ability to hold and process information significantly improves when their phones aren't near them. A 2013

Are You Addicted to Technology?

Are you anxious when you can't use your phone, computer, or device, even if it's only for a short period of time? When you do have free time, do you spend more time on your phone, computer, or device than you do engaging in hobbies or spending time with friends or family? Do you sleep with your phone or computer powered on and near your bed, checking it right before you go to bed and first thing in the morning? Do you often ignore what's happening around you because you're too absorbed in what's happening on a screen? If you answered yes to any of these questions, you may have a problem with technology. For a more thorough analysis, head to the Center for Internet and Technology Addiction website and take its fifteen-question online analysis where you'll answer inquiries like, "Do you find yourself spending more time texting, tweeting, or emailing as opposed to talking in person?" and "Do you find yourself mindlessly checking your cell or smartphone many times a day, even when you know there is likely nothing new or important to see?" If you discover or think you do have a problem, consider talking with your doctor, a psychologist, or a therapist who understands technology addiction. There are also self-help books, courses, and support groups, some of which are online—if you can, experts advise finding help off the Internet so that you don't exacerbate the dependency.

study from researchers at McGill University discovered that people who regularly depend on a smartphone or device with GPS to navigate instead of their own spatial abilities have less activity and gray matter in the hippocampus. Other research still shows that people who use the Internet the most often have difficulty focusing and discerning fact from fiction. Researchers say smartphones also prevent us from daydreaming, thinking creatively, solving problems, and having those *aha!* moments that can lead to life-changing success or happiness.

Your Phone Is Sabotaging Your Social Life

While the idea that our devices can cause social isolation isn't surprising per se, the degree to which phones are sabotaging our social lives and overall happiness is profound. Even a short stint of cell phone use can make you less likely to want to spend time with others or help friends and family, studies show. That's because researchers say our smartphones can falsely trick our brains into thinking our need for social interaction has already been met because we texted, emailed, or interacted with someone on social media.

According to the Pew Research Center, 89 percent of people use cell phones during social situations, even though 82 percent admit doing so impedes their conversation and social enjoyment. A 2018 study from researchers at the University of British Columbia also showed that people who leave their phones on the table during dinner are less likely to enjoy their company (or their meal). People who phub, or snub their friends, family members, and colleagues by using their phones in social situations, are perceived by others to be selfish and rude, while spouses and significant others say they are less satisfied in their romantic relationships with those who are on their phones too often.

Our smartphones have also become social security blankets, allowing us to bury ourselves in our devices instead of interacting with others in social situations. This, in turn, thwarts the development or growth of social skills, especially in teens and young adults, and prevents us from making new friends, business contacts, and love interests.

Technology Can Make You Anxious, Stressed, Lonely, and Even Depressed

People who spend hours daily on phones and other devices are more likely to experience a greater degree of isolation, loneliness, depression, anxiety, and suicidal thoughts than those who use technology more mindfully. Our brains and bodies, scientists say, were never designed to stare at screens for hours on end, sacrificing time we might otherwise spend with friends and family, working, cooking, exercising, enjoying the outdoors, or even daydreaming, which is critical to our overall mental and emotional health.

One study published in 2018 in the journal *Emotion* that was conducted on one million American teens found that those who spent the least amount of time in front of screens were significantly happier than those who spent the most time texting, on social media, video chatting, surfing the web, and playing video games. Every additional activity that involved a screen increased unhappiness, researchers found, with those spending more than five hours daily on screens being twice as likely to be unhappy as those who spent less than an hour per day.

Smartphones also add stress to our lives in unique ways. Devices allow people to stay connected 24/7, which isn't a good thing: this constant stream of information, potential correspondence and news, whether important or trivial, boosts stress levels dramatically, researchers have found. But because of this continual flow of information and news, being without your phone, even for a few minutes, can spike anxiety and FOMO (fear of missing out). In fact, a 2017 study from researchers at California State University shows that not being able to answer a phone call or text can send some people into stress overload.

Social media like Facebook and Instagram also trigger us to compare ourselves with others, even if what we're seeing is only what users want to show us, which is often representative of the ideal, not the norm. This comparison can cause feelings of inadequacy, low self-worth, and even depression.

Smartphones Can Make You Look Older Overnight

Turns out, looking online for the best antiaging cream or serum isn't the best way to turn back the clock: a 2018 study published in *Oxidative Medicine and Cellular Longevity* shows cell phones can prematurely age skin cells by emitting a high-energy light that accelerates skin aging—scary stuff for anyone who stares at her phone for hours every day.

That's not all: heavy cell phone users can also develop "tech neck," the term for wrinkling induced by spending hours cocked over a phone, which causes creases to form in the thin skin of the neck. Squinting at small text on a phone can also stimulate fine lines in the delicate skin around the eyes and forehead.

If you put your phone to your cheek to speak, the device's heat can boost your skin's production of melanin, a pigment that can lead to spot discoloration. Finally, a 2010 study from researchers at the University of Arizona found that cell phones can harbor ten times more bacteria than a toilet seat, which isn't good for your skin or your overall health. For your face, though, it can mean breakouts and increased acne whenever you talk without a headset.

The Sneaky Ways Technology Steals Sleep

Nearly all modern devices with a screen, like cell phones, computers, iPads, e-readers, and televisions, transmit a type of wavelength called blue light, which interferes with the body's natural sleep-wake cycle, preventing us from falling asleep and staying there. Then there's the addictive nature of technology: studies show people who use computers and smartphones before bed are much more likely to stay up later and jeopardize getting a proper night's sleep than those who disconnect earlier. As I know from personal experience, checking your email, news feed, or social media before bed can cause you to see information that energizes, stresses, or disturbs you, causing your mind to race when it should be relaxing. And if you're one of the 70 percent of Americans who sleeps with your phone by your bed and you don't power it off, then you could be woken up at night by a beep, ping, buzz, or chime.

Forget Low Carb: How Going Device-Free Can Help You Lose Weight

It may seem surprising that a device could be associated with weight gain, but our laptops, computers, and cell phones aren't just simple gadgets—they interfere with and control how we live our lives. For example, being addicted to your phone or laptop can cause stress and prevent you from getting proper sleep, both of which can contribute to weight gain. Several studies also show people are more likely to overeat and make unhealthier food choices when they're using phones or other technology, even just to text. We're also less likely to enjoy what we eat when we're using technology, meaning we're not as sated with meals and more likely to want to keep eating to get that sense of satisfaction.

Technology doesn't just affect what you eat, it also curtails how much you move. Those who are the most addicted to tech get the least exercise, studies show. And are you that person who always takes your phone to the gym with you? Research shows people who use their phones in the gym or while jogging, biking, hiking, or walking outside are less likely to get in a heart-pumping workout—and more likely to end prematurely or rest too long answering a text or call. Similarly, technology allows us to be inherently lazy: we can send texts or call family members and colleagues instead of walking to another room to speak with them directly, order delivery from our laptops instead of cooking or making the effort to go out, and watch any show at any time instead of engaging in activities that would take us off the chair or couch.

Technology Is Wrecking Your Posture, Eyesight, and Dexterity

Why do many twenty-year-olds have the spinal health of those much older, in their thirties or forties? Chiropractors finger one primary cause: too much technology use. The problem, they say, is years of looking down at phones, which adds approximately sixty pounds of strain to your neck and back every time you do so, according to research published in 2014 in *Surgical Technology International*. Over months and years, this constant strain, along with the stance you assume when you hunch over a device, can create pain and lasting posture problems. In more severe cases, people have developed compressed discs and long-term nerve damage just by spending too much time working on computers and phones.

These devices aren't just hurting our backs, but also killing our vision by causing digital eye strain—a serious condition that affects approximately 60 percent of Americans, causing headaches, dry eyes, blurred vision, double vision, and discomfort. Symptoms can go away with reduced tech use, but some people experience lasting effects. Getting too much blue light, emitted by technology screens, also changes certain cells in our eyes, accelerating the risk of macular degeneration and even blindness, researchers say.

Finally, constantly scrolling, texting, and typing on a smartphone can cause cramped fingers, wrist pain, and inflammation throughout the hand. For this reason, several studies have found a link between phone use and carpal tunnel syndrome.

Smartphones Can Even Kill You

Traffic fatalities have increased considerably in recent years—and major organizations like the National Safety Council are blaming the bump on distracted drivers. Cell phone use now accounts for approximately 15 percent of all fatal motor-vehicle accidents, causing thousands of deaths, along with hundreds of thousands of injuries, every year. Experts at the National Highway Traffic and Safety Administration say using a phone while driving is even deadlier than getting behind the wheel after a few drinks—it takes only three seconds of looking down at your phone to cause a crash, they say, which is the time it takes for your car to cover a football field if you're driving 55 miles per hour. Of course, it's not just your safety you have to worry about: distracted drivers kill and maim other drivers, passengers, cyclists, and pedestrians—a mistake that can ruin the rest of your life.

Pedestrian deaths are also on the rise in recent years, as the number of people who walk and text has soared enormously. Whether you live in a busy city like New York, the suburbs, or a small town, you can injure yourself by not paying attention to the cars, trucks, bikes, uneven road surfaces, trees, potholes, and poles around you. The problem isn't exclusive to the streets, either: according to the National Safety Council, people are most likely to be injured due to walking and texting in their own homes, tripping over furniture and rugs or walking into unforeseen objects. For all these reasons, the council now lists "distracted walking" as one of its hazards.

AUGUST MINDFUL TECH: Your Story

Whether you're a total tech addict or think you have a good grip on your device use, limiting the amount of time you spend on computers, laptops, tablets, smartphones, and social media isn't easy.

Technology has become so widespread and universal in our lives that it's likely more intrinsic to your daily routine than you think. But perhaps the most difficult part of the challenge is figuring out the best way you, the reader, can learn to consume technology more mindfully. If you don't take long walks on a regular basis—or if you do, but aren't usually buried in your phone—my initial target to avoid my phone when walking won't help you accomplish this month's goals. That's why it's critical to address the first tip below and really take the time to discern the best way to reduce your technology consumption. Once you do that, the nine other tips listed here can help you get off your devices and start living in the real world once again.

1. TURN YOUR TECH GAZE INWARD. We all have unique work demands, daily habits, and personal preferences that dictate how and when we consume technology. For me, my biggest problem was overusing my phone—for others, it could be that you spend too much time on your computer, laptop, tablet, smartwatch, or a combination thereof. Others might have an addiction to a certain platform like social media, email, or the web. The first step to recovery is understanding the issue as it affects you, so take the time to identify where and with which device you might have a problem.

    Once you identify the problem, it can help you strategize a solution specific to your individual addiction, along with your daily routine and lifestyle. For example, if you don't walk more than five minutes at a time—or you do but would never use your phone—adopting my phone-free strolls won't help. Analyze your daily schedule to figure out the times and for which activities you can reduce or eliminate technology. Be curious and open to evolving how you choose to limit technology as the days and weeks progress. I never assumed I had the right formula that allowed me to adopt more productive habits as the month went on. At the very least, I'd encourage you to stop using your phone during meals or social events—it's not only rude but also interferes with your relationships, digestion, and overall happiness.

2.   TAKE BABY STEPS. If you know you're attached to your phone or have to use a computer all day for work, don't make it your starting mission to give up this device for hours on end. I began the month with a realistic, sustainable goal of not using my phone for thirty minutes to an hour during one activity I did most days of the week, which ensured I'd start the challenge successfully reducing my tech consumption on Day 1. In this regard, it's better to set minigoals and add objectives cumulatively than to go out of the gate with a finish line you're unlikely to ever cross. Remember, the end goal is to limit and ultimately change your dependency on technology, so any step that brings you closer to that goal is one in the right direction.

3.   TURN OFF NOTIFICATIONS. One reason we're all so addicted to our phones and computers is that they're constantly beeping, buzzing, chiming, and chirping to tell us every single time there's a new email, message, tweet, comment, news article, or completely irrelevant update. Scientists say these notifications can trigger a dopamine response, increasing the likelihood of addiction as we check our phones every few seconds to see what the unknown might hold, as well as feel as though we're more important or cared for by others or the world at large because our phones are dinging at us. The best way to end this addiction, experts say, is to simply turn off notifications except for the most important communications. You can still see what the unknown holds whenever you choose to take a look rather than only doing so when your device tells you something's important.

4.   TAKE TO HEART WHAT OTHERS SAY ABOUT YOUR TECH CON-SUMPTION. When I started the Mindful Tech Challenge, one

primary goal I wanted to accomplish was to reduce phubbing when with my kids—they had already complained about it many times over. Your friends, family members, and colleagues can also help tip you off to those habits you should try to change. For example, has anyone reprimanded you for texting or checking your phone during dinner? Have friends ever commented or joked about how much time you spend taking or posting pictures to Instagram? If no one has ever said anything to you, don't be afraid to ask for honest feedback.

5. SEE IT IN OTHERS SO YOU CAN CHANGE IT IN YOURSELF. I started paying closer attention this month to how people around me used technology, which helped me to make some startling conclusions about my own behaviors. For example, when I wasn't always on my own phone, I began to notice how rude it was for others to text, email, or take calls when out at restaurants and bars—and how clearly annoyed their dates, spouses, friends, or family were when they did this. I also started to see people dangerously close to accidents while walking and texting, and how inconsiderate it was to the other pedestrians, cyclists, and even drivers who had to navigate around them. I began to feel sorry for people who couldn't silence their phones during concerts, lectures, or conference meetings, or who seemed more concerned with capturing a moment or event for social media than enjoying that moment or event themselves. Becoming more aware of how others use technology can make you recognize these behaviors in yourself and motivate you to change those habits you don't respect in others.

6. GET COMFORTABLE WITH BEING UNCOMFORTABLE. Most people are accustomed to being constantly stimulated by a device. Whenever we have free time, like when we have to wait for a train, elevator, friend, or appointment, we scroll,

stare at, and mindlessly interact with our phones or computers. Stopping this habit to allow your mind to entertain itself can be uncomfortable at first, making you feel bored or useless, or causing you to consider issues in your life you'd rather ignore. But this is exactly what technology addiction experts say we need to do: spend time with ourselves, in our own minds, daydreaming, working through our problems, and, most important, learning to be comfortable with who we are and how we feel. Try to endure the initial boredom or discomfort you might feel when not on a device. Doing so can ultimately make you happier and more comfortable in your own skin than you've ever been.

7. TELL YOUR COLLEAGUES, FRIENDS, AND FAMILY YOU'RE GOING OFF THE GRID. I had an easier time disconnecting while on vacation when I set an out-of-office reply—this way, I was assured neither my colleagues nor my patients would be expecting or waiting for a response. I also told my friends, kids, and parents about the challenge so they knew that whenever I was out to dinner, taking a walk, or on vacation, I wouldn't be available by text or email and that they should call only if there was a dire emergency. Taking these steps went a long way to reducing the number of gratuitous texts, calls, and emails I received during the month. Furthermore, whenever I was with my colleagues, friends, and family, I was less likely to use my phone because they all knew I was doing the challenge and I'd look silly if I did. Bottom line: While I've said it about nearly every challenge to date, sharing your month's mission with everyone you know can help ensure your success in more ways than one.

8. REMEMBER THAT TEXTS AND EMAILS ARE BILATERAL IN THE CYBERSPHERE. If you don't like to be texted or emailed about non-life-threatening issues late at night, early in the

morning, or on the weekends, don't do the same to your colleagues, friends, and family. Being mindful of how you use
technology extends to how you ask others to consume technology, too. If you're sending a text just to say hi or let someone know you're thinking about them, consider a different
type of communication that might relay this message more
meaningfully, like a written note or a phone call.

9. SET YOUR PHONE TO DO NOT DISTURB AT NIGHT. There's no
   reason you need to wake up at every text, email, and social
   media alert in the overnight hours. After all, are you really
   going to respond? Instead, set your phone to Do Not Disturb.
   In this mode, your phone will still receive texts, emails, calls,
   and other messages, but it won't illuminate, vibrate, or make
   noises, all of which can wake you up. If you're concerned
   about missing an emergency text or call from family or
   work, program "favorites" numbers into your phone, which
   will allow you to still receive calls and messages from those
   contacts in the Do Not Disturb setting.

10. DO IT TO SAVE A LIFE. I didn't choose to take phone-free
    walks because I knew I was being unsafe. But as soon as I
    started, I began to realize how much I was putting my life in
    peril on a near-daily basis by walking with my phone. Walk-
    ing or driving while texting injures and kills thousands of
    people every year. If you do either, you're putting your life
    and the lives of others at risk every day—it's also a sign you
    likely have a problem with technology. If you don't do this
    challenge for any other reason, do it to save a life, which may
    even be your own.

9

SEPTEMBER

Less Sugar

My Story

Sugar—it's what's for dinner, literally and figuratively. Not only are Americans consuming more sweet stuff than we ever have before, we're also now barraged with the news of just how detrimental too much sugar is for our hearts, brains, bodies, and overall physical, mental, and emotional health. The harm of excessive dietary sugar is a subject that just doesn't go away. As a doctor, nutritionist, and on-air medical correspondent, I talk about it every day with patients and seem to do a segment on some facet of sugar at least once a month for *GMA*. That said, I knew I couldn't write this book without challenging myself and thousands of others to reduce our daily sugar consumption.

I'll admit, though, that I'm lucky. At baseline, I don't have a sweet tooth. I rarely eat sugar, mostly because I avoid nearly all the processed carbs that contain it. But I also don't crave sweet things and almost never eat dessert, in part because I have food allergies that prevent me from enjoying many traditional sweets. Before this month began, if you asked me to grade my sugar consumption, I would have given myself a B+. Whenever I'd calculated my daily sugar intake in the past, I was usually far below twenty-five grams of added sugar, which is what the World Health Organization (WHO) recommends women don't exceed per day. (Men, those lucky guys, are allowed slightly more sweet stuff, at thirty-eight grams per day.)

Despite the fact I felt I was doing well in the sugar department, I wanted to see if I could curtail my total and added sugar intake even more and bring my overall consumption up to an A+—that's how strongly I feel about limiting our sugar intake for our overall health. I was also curious to see whether cutting out nearly all sugar would affect my energy levels and the constant skin blotchiness I loathe, in addition to seeing whether it would help me lose body fat and belly bloat. I decided I'd make it my monthly goal to make sure I was at or below the WHO's suggestion of no more than twenty-five grams of added sugar per day.

What are added sugars? Flip over the package of nearly any processed foods, and they tend to be somewhere in the ingredient list, disguised under the names of sucrose, fructose, glucose, dextrose, lactose, maltose, corn syrup, brown rice syrup, and dozens of other different varieties, along with natural sources like fruit, fruit juice, honey, maple syrup, agave, molasses, and fruit juice concentrates added to sweeten foods and beverages. Added sugars are found in the majority of processed food, even ones that aren't sweet per se like spaghetti sauce, salad dressing, yogurt, cereal, and protein bars. These added sugars are different from naturally occurring sugars found in whole grains, dairy, legumes, and even vegetables, which do not negatively impact health and are not factored into the WHO's daily recommendations.

Before this challenge, I consumed the majority of my daily added sugar from foods like packaged Greek yogurt, which can contain a lot, along with condiments like ketchup, salad dressing, and honey that I'd drizzle over sliced banana and a Wasa cracker. I also factored into my sugar count any glasses of wine I had and the ever-occasional *affogato,* or vanilla ice cream topped with espresso, that I'd order on a special occasion if eating out.

The only exception to my seemingly angelic sugar consumption— and it's a sizable one—is cookies/brownies, especially the homemade kind. They're my weakness, especially since Chloe likes to bake both whenever she's home from boarding school. When she does, and she's quite skilled at it, I impulsively and compulsively eat them around the clock until they're gone. For this reason, I never keep cookies or brownies at home when she's not, and I try to encourage her to give her goodies to friends in the city or take them back to school with her. But I decided not to worry about the threat of cookies and brownies this month—I could control myself if I tried, and since I had a challenge to complete, I assumed I'd be able to steer clear of temptation for thirty days. In fact, overall, I felt confident this month's challenge would be a piece of cake.

Week 1
The Incredible Influence of Sugar on Cravings and Self-Control

My new mission this month was clear: read labels and count sugar grams in everything I ate, staying at or below twenty-five grams at all times. The target of this month and way to measure it were so clear—no ambiguity or devising a means to meet my goals like I struggled with during my Mindful Tech Challenge. And since I had no trepidation about my potential success, the week started well: I had no problem staying below twenty-five grams daily. Things were going wonderfully, in fact, until the third day, when I went to a family gathering at my father's apartment. I was enjoying his company and not even thinking about the challenge when my son, Alex, walked in with chocolate chip cookies from famed New York City pastry chef Jacques Torres.

If you've never had a Jacques Torres cookie, you haven't experienced cookie completeness. Picture giant, freshly baked discs of deliciousness, each cookie the size of a medium pancake, with absolutely no ingredients to which I'm allergic. When I saw my son walk in with a bag, my first thought was, *I'm screwed.*

After dinner ended and the cookies were brought out in all their aromatic glory, I felt like a dog who had a steak dropped on the floor in front of me. I subconsciously felt the challenge go out the back of my brain. I broke off a half and tried in vain to nibble on it, but soon, that half become the whole. I felt like an addict, entirely powerless over my vice. I started laughing and shaking my head at the same time: this was Day 3 of the month and I was already blowing my added sugar consumption for nearly the week. And I couldn't even blame the slipup on a glass of wine or tequila—I was too careful about my drinking now to waste one of my seven servings on a night when I was trying to eat well. My only consolation was that we didn't take any cookies home, because if we had, I would have not been able to stop.

I was able to get back on track momentarily, but near the end of the week, that track derailed again. Chloe was home again from school, and I talked myself into buying her an oversize bar of dark chocolate after reading a study that said the high concentration of cocoa helps with muscle recovery. This was a clear case of rationalization: she doesn't buy herself chocolate or even necessarily like dark chocolate. At the same time, I knew the research on recovery was just as strong for healthier foods like salmon and plain yogurt. But I wanted that chocolate. It was calling my name.

Before she even got home, I had opened the bar and, despite telling myself I'd only have one square, consumed an entire half—and this was bigger than a normal candy bar, too. I wasn't even a chocolate hound, but here I was, bizarrely devouring the bar as though it was all I had ever craved. This month was supposed to be easy, I had thought, but not even a full week in and I'd already consumed more sugar than I normally would for an entire month. The reason, I knew, was the deprivation effect I'd already experienced at the start of other challenges, like during my dry month and when I tried to cut out red meat. But this time, the pull of sugar felt stronger, and I began to doubt just how successful I'd be at overcoming a sweets addiction.

At the week's end, I felt like a failure. Instead of completing one-fourth of the challenge feeling cleaner and leaner like I had after the Hydration; Less Meat, More Plants; and Cardio Challenges, I was seven days into blah and more bloated. Sure, I'd had only one giant cookie and half of a massive chocolate bar, but these weren't foods I even ate regularly when I wasn't doing a sugar challenge—and certainly weren't the ones that would catapult me to that A+ grade I was dreaming of giving myself! I even considered whether I should just start the challenge over again, pretending Week 2 was Week 1. But I decided failure was part of the experiment, and the only thing to do was get back on the wagon.

Week 2
The Secret Sugar Addiction You May Not Even Know About

The second week, I was determined to get back to my low-sugar baseline where I didn't crave cookies or chocolate. For the entire workweek, I was successful, too, and began to feel better, physically and mentally. *See, last week was just an odd aberration. I can do this!* I thought to myself. That was all before I got on a plane on Friday to go to a hockey tournament for Chloe in Canada over the weekend.

Youth sporting weekends aren't particularly renowned for healthy eating options—they're often replete with lots of pub food, processed protein bars, and sugary sports drinks, all of which is fine for high-performing high school athletes in moderation. Knowing this in advance, I'm usually able to navigate games, tournaments, and tailgating parties while maintaining my low-carb, high-plant diet, trying to keep in mind the healthy swaps I made during

May's Less Meat, More Plants Challenge. But in this instance—
and during a sugar challenge, of all times—I had no such luck in
keeping sugar out of the evening.

After dinner on tournament night, Chloe wanted ice cream. This
isn't a trigger food for me like cookies and brownies are, but the
shop she suggested was known around the world for having some of
the best homemade ice cream this side of the Atlantic. As we waited
in line, I had the opportunity to see dozens of delectable-looking
cones and cups, and I could feel my mouth begin to water. I couldn't
take it anymore by the time we got to the counter, and I ordered a
kid-size cup of cookies and cream with extra Oreo crumbles. The
dessert wasn't crazy in size or scope, but I was surprised how much
I wanted it—and subsequently enjoyed it, without a single drop of
guilt. What I felt instead was a bit incredulous I was continuing
to eat sugar—and not just more Greek yogurt or granola bars but
sugary desserts, nonetheless—in a month when I was supposed to
be doing the exact opposite.

There's one explainer here I want to make: during an ordinary
month, when you're not trying to complete a low-sugar challenge, I
don't think there's anything wrong with enjoying sweets at special
places or on special occasions. In fact, I encourage patients, even
those who want to lose weight, to indulge in the occasional treat
when and if it presents itself—otherwise you can feel deprived and
set yourself up for failure.

In this instance, I was in a foreign country with my daughter at
a place known internationally for its desserts—it wasn't as though
we were at the ice cream shop across from our apartment on a Tues-
day night. In addition, I hadn't detoured the team there or even
suggested to Chloe we go: I was simply participating in the weekend's activities, and, objectively, it should have been no big deal.
But it was a big deal this time around, because I felt like I was
unable to say no to sugar now—a problem I'd never encountered
before. I had no problem saying no to alcohol over and over again

during my dry month, but this was an addiction. And it was about to get worse.

The next day, after we were back in the city, Alex brought home a bag of Tate's Bake Shop Chocolate Chip Cookies. I didn't even hesitate, consuming one within a minute of the bag entering the apartment. And then, since they're relatively small and thin, I decided I could eat two more.

That's when I began physically to feel the effects of two weeks of consuming more concentrated sugar than I normally do: I was lethargic, bloated, and even a little nauseated. But worse still, I wanted more dessert. Despite feeling so poorly, I was craving sugar. Later that night, I even hunted around the kitchen for extra cookies or something, anything that would satisfy what seemed to be a developing sweet tooth.

At the end of the week, I wasn't just disappointed, I was also angry at myself for failing so miserably. In fourteen days, I had had more desserts—not just sugar but actual dessert—than I'd consumed in months. I began to wonder whether I was unlocking some hidden sweet tooth inside me by doing the challenge. It was becoming such an extreme 180-degree reversal that it almost felt laughable.

I also now realized I should have told those around me that I was on a Less Sugar Challenge, like I did during the Dry Challenge in January: it would have made me accountable and also lessened the likelihood of Chloe or Alex showing up to two occasions with my favorite dessert. The bigger realization, though, was how truly addicting sugar can be. Like most people, I had never thought a sugar dependency could be as powerful as an addiction to drugs, alcohol, cigarettes, gambling, or other well-known vices. Our society, in commercials, movies, music, and other cultural references, pokes fun at or even celebrates sugar cravings and overeating. But I was discovering the addiction was very real, with real consequences. I no longer felt so confident going into the third week.

Week 3

How Your Failures Can Teach You as Much as Your Successes

A pattern was now starting to emerge, as I learned I could stick to my low-sugar diet if I didn't stray from my work-life routine. For the start of the week, like the week prior, I was too busy with *GMA*, patients, and my gym routine, without any travel or special occasions to tempt me from my low-sugar resolve. That said, I still couldn't shake what seemed to be a newfound sweet tooth. One night, while working on a *GMA* segment after dinner, I felt myself starting to crave something sugary. I tried to distract myself with some planks and push-ups, which I found are a great way to keep yourself from mindless eating at night. But this time, they didn't work, so I talked myself into having the healthy "sweet" snack that normally satisfies my sugar desire—a sliced banana on Wasa with honey. But I was surprised how powerful and quickly my cravings now came.

Toward the end of the week, my routine unexpectedly went awry when I stopped quickly into my office to pick up paperwork. My nurse was also unexpectedly there—and unexpectedly happened to have some Tate's cookies, only because I had raved about them the week before. And similar to the week before, I couldn't resist, eating two before I started to find the paperwork that had brought me to the office in the first place.

By this time in the month, I knew something was seriously wrong—and I had to start taking serious action. I asked her to take the cookies home with her and never bring them into the office again. We've been working together for fourteen years, so she knew my request had nothing to do with her—and everything to do with my intent to eat healthfully. We'd also done the same thing every year around the holidays, ridding the office of the cookies, pies, chocolate, and other treats patients often sent—what we had jokingly come to refer to as "sabotage." On this night, all I asked her to do was simply remove the "sabotage" from my sight for the foreseeable future. Making this adamant request made me feel better. I also resolved to make sure I meditated every morning of Week 3 and drank more water—two techniques I now knew would help stabilize my appetite from my challenges earlier in the year. Finally, I felt like I was being proactive about the challenge, not just acting incredulous about my failures.

That weekend, I traveled to Boston to visit my boyfriend, and the first night, we ate with friends at one of my favorite restaurants in the city. At most places, I don't risk ordering dessert because I don't trust it won't contain an ingredient to which I'm allergic. But I'd been to this restaurant many times before and knew they had these small cinnamon-sugar doughnuts that were entirely allergy-friendly. In my head, I already made the same rationalization I had in the Canadian ice cream shop: I was out with friends at my favorite restaurant on a weekend excursion and enjoying a mini-doughnut was an intrinsic and inevitable part of the experience. Thankfully, I only had one, but that now didn't matter so much—the feelings of failure came rushing back.

Now I knew that at the end of the month, I would have to look at myself in the mirror and tell myself I had failed the Less Sugar Challenge. It was my first failure to date, and while unpleasant, I also knew I was learning more than I would be if I had been successful. For example, I would have never realized just how powerful sugar addictions and sugar cravings could be, and I wouldn't have ever developed empathy for patients who suffer these kinds of cravings on an hourly basis. I would have never learned the physical effects consuming too much added sugar can cause, making you feel lethargic, irritable, incredibly bloated, and nauseated, yet still hungry for more.

I looked back at my arrogance at the beginning of the month and realized how wrong I had been. Anyone can be addicted to sugar, and I had always been—I just hadn't been aware of how much sugar I was consuming in the past. I had mistakenly thought I could control sugar cravings, but I was now learning the addiction can be overwhelming, if not crippling. For these reasons, I decided to continue to try to eat less sugar the next month and that, feelings of failure aside, I had to try to finish the week without any slipups.

Week 4
How to Lose Your Sweet Tooth and Kick Sugar for Good

You can replay the record of the last few weeks, and this week, the song would have been the same. Despite my new resolve, I cracked midweek after a patient brought dark chocolate to the office. Since she had given it to me under the auspices of being healthy, that's also how I viewed it: a beneficial treat I didn't eat enough of. I ate half the bar.

Afterward, I felt racked by disappointment and doubt. This was the last week, the one I'd resolved to have nothing get in the way of some success. Yet here I was, unable to control my urges and scarfing down dessert like it was kale. Thankfully, this was my only slip for the week.

As the month came to a close, though, I knew I had completely failed the challenge, but succeeded in learning more about myself than I had in any other month. This had proved to me what this book is all about: self-experimentation. By experimenting, I learned I possessed just as much of a sweet tooth as anyone else, one I'd never been conscious of before but that was still there, feeding a vicious cycle of cravings and consumption that eventually becomes an addiction. By the last week, I felt powerless over sugar: if I was offered a cookie or chocolate, I would have to eat it, regardless of my level of determination, commitment, or resolve. And while one kiddie cup of ice cream or a small sugar doughnut may seem harmless in itself, I also now knew a concentrated dose of added sugar on any scale would awaken my sweet tooth and trigger cravings I couldn't control.

I also realized I was more successful with an all-or-nothing approach when it came to sweet treats. This strategy was key, after all, to my dry month—had I allowed myself only a glass or two of wine per week, I think I would have likely given myself permission to have more here or there when I wanted. Similarly, at the beginning of the month, I had wrongly assumed I could just nibble at a cookie or have a single chocolate square. But while others may be able to do this, I couldn't—I either needed to avoid it completely or accept the possibility I'd eat more than I bargained for. Some people thrive on the three-bite rule, where they enjoy only a few bites of a food before putting it down, but I learned I can't do that with desserts, despite what I tell myself.

Perhaps most important, I learned what it's like to fail. I had never crashed and burned so much in a challenge to date but doing so taught me two major lessons. First, I learned how to forgive myself: failing at something didn't make me a failure—I was still myself and wonderful in all the ways that make me *me* (cue the personal pep talk music!). Second, since I had failed but still continued to keep trying, starting each week with fresh resolve, I had learned how to persevere. And learning to persevere allowed me to continue my sugar challenge into October, taking all the lessons I'd learned in September so that I had a better chance at success. Sometimes, it takes a little more time to figure out the best ways to approach a challenge—I learned that in August when I struggled to find different ways to use my phone more mindfully. And you have to make mistakes first so you can learn the ways to avoid them before you're able to adopt a new health habit.

For the next thirty days, I consumed only one forkful of dessert—and that only because my daughter begged me to try something after she accompanied me on a work trip to Europe. This was less added sugar than I had had in years. Finally, I had completed the sugar washout I had hoped for last month. As a result, I answered the questions I had hoped to: my skin looked less red, I had more energy, I was less bloated, and I had lost body fat. But most important, I had lost my sweet tooth.

SEPTEMBER LESS SUGAR:
The Science Behind Consuming Less Sugar

Reducing how much added sugar you eat has so many benefits to your brain and body that enumerating them all would take up an entire book in itself. And if you're interested, those books have already been written, many times over. But giving up sugar has some surprising benefits many don't know, along with advantages I found interesting in my journey to discover a healthier way to interact with America's number one addiction.

Sugar Can Be Just as Addictive as Street Drugs

While some question whether food can really be addictive, the research on how sugar affects the brain doesn't vary in its conclusions. Study after study shows sugar can have the same effect on the brain as many street drugs, activating the same area of the brain and triggering a similar cycle of highs, lows, cravings, binges, and withdrawal.

According to Dr. Nicole Avena, who has led most of the top research on sugar addiction, eating sweet stuff stimulates the brain's reward system, also activated by drugs, sex, and love, triggering a release of dopamine that creates feelings of pleasure and happiness. And similar to drugs, sugar can also overactivate this reward system, causing severe cravings and a loss of control. The more you consume, the more you want and need to get the same surge of dopamine, just like drugs. Over time, your cravings intensify, and when you don't eat sugar, you don't feel happy—although by now, you need so much sugar to feel happy, you have to eat an entire bag of Tate's cookies to get the same dopamine response you used to get from one cookie. For all these reasons, Dr. Avena's research has shown rats will take Oreos over cocaine if given the choice—that's how addictive sugar can be.

You're Eating Way More Sugar Than You Think

Three-quarters of packaged foods on supermarket shelves today, including savory items, contain added sugar. Chances are, in fact, if you're eating something out of a package, carton, wrapper, bottle, or box, it contains added sugar. For these reasons, the average American consumes eighty-two grams of sugar per day—fifty-seven grams more than the World Health Organization's daily maximum for women—totaling sixty-six *pounds* of added sugar per person per year. Many foods you'd never suspect contain added sugar, including yogurt, sushi, tomato sauce, bread, nut butters, salad dressings, instant oatmeal, cereal, beef jerky, and granola and protein bars. If you're skeptical, take a look at the nutrition labels of your favorite packaged foods. You'll likely be shocked by how much sugar is in a single serving.

Sugar Can Age You and Wreck Your Skin

If the health benefits alone don't convince you to cut sugar, then maybe vanity will. While everyone knows spending too much time in the sun can cause discoloration and fine lines, few realize that eating too much sugar can produce the exact same effects. That's because sugar bonds to collagen and other proteins in our skin, causing cells to stiffen and become less elastic. Over time, this creates the appearance of fine lines, spots, and sagging, as excess sugar eventually damages cell collagen and elastin. Eating too much sweet stuff can also cause acne by weakening our immune response while boosting testosterone, which widens pores and stimulates oil production. And we haven't even begun to detail how sugar has been associated with chronic inflammation and weight gain, both of which can ruin skin health.

Sugar Sabotages Your Smarts

Your brain needs sugar to subsist—this is fundamental biochemistry. But eat too much, as the majority of us do, and it will slow your mental processes and make you less able to learn new information and recall facts. In fact, a 2012 animal study from researchers at UCLA found that six weeks of a high-sugar diet—that is, what the average American eats—is all it takes to impede cognitive function. Researchers have also found a link between sugar consumption and cognitive diseases like Alzheimer's and dementia. Some doctors even refer to Alzheimer's as "type 3 diabetes," or a condition brought on in part by elevated blood sugar and subsequent insulin resistance.

Don't Drown Your Problems in Ice Cream—It'll Make Everything Worse

The common remedy for a bad breakup or a rough day at the office may be some Ben & Jerry's, but eating this kind of added sugar won't make you feel anything but more anxiety, moodiness, and even depression. Although it's true the sugar in Chubby Hubby or a candy bar can trigger a release of mood-boosting dopamine, similar to what happens when we drink alcohol, these good feelings eventually come crashing down, as that happiness high eventually turns into lethargy, irritability, fatigue, and brain fog. Researchers have even found that consuming too much sugar can contribute to clinical depression.

Sugar Can Ruin Your Teeth and Make Your Breath Smell Bad

You likely already know sugary foods can cause cavities. But that's not all the sweet stuff does to your oral health. Sugar is a direct cause of gum disease, raising the acidity in your mouth and feeding bad bacteria that attack teeth and gums. This bad bacteria can also cause foul breath, multiplying so quickly that no amount of gum or toothpaste can counter your malodorous mouth. If that's not shocking enough, this surplus of bad bacteria can also escape into your bloodstream, increasing your risk of heart disease, dementia, and rheumatoid arthritis, among other serious ailments.

Sugar Raises the Risk of Heart Disease, Cancer, and Other Chronic Disease

A number of studies show people who eat or drink more sugar have an associated higher incidence of heart attack and heart disease than those who consume less. In fact, a 2018 report from an American Heart Association study found people who drink twenty-four ounces or more of sugary beverages per day have double the risk of dying from heart disease than those who drink less than one ounce daily. Conclusive evidence also links sugar consumption to an elevated risk of type 2 diabetes and fatty liver disease. This relationship is based on both association and causation—the holy grail for science and medicine—meaning the more sugar you eat, the more you'll undoubtedly and inevitably increase your chances of incurring both conditions.

As for cancer, while researchers haven't yet been able to conclusively link sugar consumption to an increased risk, the existing evidence is enough to make anyone reconsider eating a whole bag of cookies. A nine-year study published in 2017 in *Nature Communications* demonstrates a link between glucose consumption and cancer progression, meaning sugar may literally help feed cancer cells, causing them to multiply and do so more rapidly. Researchers also say sugar increases the risk of being overweight or obese, both of which raise cancer risk exponentially.

SEPTEMBER LESS SUGAR: Your Story

I learned the hard way that reducing sugar in your diet isn't easy. Sugar cravings are legitimate and intense, a fact many restaurants and food manufacturers already know. That's why sugar can be found in three-quarters of all packaged foods and in the majority of prepared meals and sides you'll find at restaurants, grocery stores, fast-casual chains, and fast-food shops. This list doesn't exclude seemingly "healthy" items like salads, smoothies, quinoa cups, and acai bowls, all of which research shows can contain excessive amounts of added sweeteners. Still, cutting down on your added sugar intake isn't impossible by any means—you just need to learn a few tricks of the trade. Here are the ten I found most useful in the two months total I tried to cut my added sugar intake.

1. PUT IN SOME PREP TIME. The month will be far more difficult if your kitchen harbors cookies, cakes, candy, ice cream, or any other traditional desserts in general. But it'll also be nearly impossible if your home is stocked with processed foods also high in sugar, items like cereal, granola bars, fruit-flavored yogurt, commercial salad dressings, and other foods that contain just as much sugar as traditional desserts. Before you begin, do yourself a favor and donate your sugary foods to a local soup kitchen or homeless shelter. If your spouse or kids object, tell them they can still eat sweets outside the house, but can't bring them inside for thirty days.

   After you've made your kitchen a safe space, do the same for your office, home work space, car, and purse. If you keep stashes of candies or sugary protein bars in these places, give them away or donate them. The less temptation in your home and work spaces, the more likely you will be able to succeed.

2. TELL EVERYONE. If I could do my initial low-sugar month all over again, the first thing I would do is tell everyone I was on a Less Sugar Challenge. This would have created accountability for me and made it less likely my friends, family, colleagues, and patients would offer me irresistible cookies, chocolate, and other desserts. Don't wait for the right moment or for sugar to make an appearance in your relationships: tell your nearest and dearest before the month even begins so they can help you thwart temptation before temptation suddenly thwarts you.

3. LEARN TO READ LABELS. If there's one relatively easy thing about this challenge, it's that the nutrition labels on packaged foods and drinks now make understanding your added sugar intake as easy as apple pie, no pun intended. As of the end of 2018, the FDA now requires most food sold in bags, boxes, and wrappers to list how many grams of added sugar they contain in a separate, designated line. Just scan the nutrition label until you see the "Added Sugars" line beneath "Total Sugars." If you don't see this information, take a look at the "Sugars" under "Carbohydrates"—this tells how many sugar grams total a product contains, both natural and added. Unless your food contains primarily whole fruit, vegetables, and grains (with the word *whole* before any grain), the Sugars line can be a good indicator of how many added sugar grams that food or drink contains.

4. TRACK TWENTY-FIVE (OR THIRTY-EIGHT) GRAMS ANY WAY YOU CAN. Throughout the month, I remained very aware of the number twenty-five—the maximum number of added

sugar grams the World Health Organization recommends women consume daily (the maximum number for men is thirty-eight grams). The days I didn't slip up with cookies, chocolate, ice cream, or doughnuts, I stayed at or below this number. While I found it easy to keep track of added sugar in my head, if you're not used to analyzing how much sugar you eat daily—and most people aren't—keep a tally of your added sugar intake in the notes on your phone or in a notebook you keep in your purse. There are also apps for your phone that can track added sugar for you. Try Fooducate, which provides the added sugar amount in over 250,000 grocery items, or Wholesome, which can track your total sugar intake and warns you when you've had too much. Just remember to accurately input your serving size, which most people underestimate.

5. CHOOSE UNPROCESSED FOODS FOR EASY, SIMPLE SUCCESS. Whole, unprocessed foods like fresh vegetables, whole fruit from the produce section, fresh seafood, chicken and beef, dry beans and legumes, grains you cook yourself, and plain dairy with nothing added don't contain added sugars. That means you don't have to worry about reading labels or tracking sugar grams when you choose whole, unprocessed foods. But be skeptical of anything you buy in a box, bag, carton, or wrapper: many deli meats, flavored dairy foods, boxed or bagged grains, and frozen or bagged products that may appear to be made from mostly vegetables or fruit still harbor hidden sugar. Read the ingredient list and scan the label if you're unsure.

6. HAVE A BACKUP STRATEGY FOR YOUR SWEET TOOTH. Another action I wish I had taken before my less sugar month was to find substitutions that would stand in for desserts at family dinners and other special occasions. If I had had a

go-to low-sugar dessert alternative already in place, like fresh strawberries with balsamic vinegar, I would have brought this to the family dinner at my father's where my first slip occurred. That way, I could still have enjoyed a treat and felt like I wasn't depriving myself but wouldn't have added a single gram of added sugar to my daily total.

Other low-sugar alternatives include plain yogurt with cacao nibs (these crunchy bits taste like chocolate but contain no added sugar); frozen grapes or bananas; fruit salad; protein or food bars that contain no added sugar; baked apples or poached pears with toasted nuts; and after-dinner coffee or tea with milk and cinnamon. If you're the type more tempted by salty sweets like chocolate-dipped pretzels or pecan pie, try popcorn tossed with olive oil and cinnamon or caramelized vegetables served with ginger or nutmeg.

7. UNDERSTAND IT TAKES TIME TO RETRAIN TASTE BUDS. If you consume lots of processed sugar on a daily basis, cutting back to 25 or 38 grams daily will be difficult at first. But studies show you can retrain your taste buds within a few weeks' time. That means that if you're persistent about slowly cutting back on sugar, midway through the month, you may find foods begin to taste too sweet or that your coffee is good with only one packet of sugar instead of two. To this extent, research shows children can begin to like foods they thought they didn't after only one single bite. Scientists say adults can adapt similarly, beginning to enjoy foods like unsweetened yogurt, cereal, salad dressing, and sauces after eating them only three or four times.

8. TARGET LOW-HANGING FRUIT. Sugary beverages like soda, fancy coffee drinks, shakes, smoothies, and energy drinks are the most concentrated (read: worst) sources of added sugar you can consume. Not only do most sugary drinks

contain ridiculous amounts of added sugar—a medium-size flavored latte can easily top your maximum daily intake, while a small-size smoothie may double your per diem—they don't contain the fat, protein, or fiber you need to slow that sugar from rushing straight into your bloodstream, causing an insulin spike that leads to lethargy, bad mood, increased appetite, and weight gain. The solution: drop the sugary drinks from your diet as soon as you can. This will do more to reduce your cravings than any other single change. Plus, there are now hundreds of options that make ditching sweet drinks easier than ever. Think unsweetened, flavored seltzer instead of soda, unsweetened cappuccino or high-quality espresso in lieu of pumpkin-spice anything, or a piece of real fruit instead of a juice smoothie.

9. TAKE IT SERIOUSLY. Sugar addiction is real—and can have devastating consequences on physical, mental, and emotional health. I wish I had understood just how powerful sugar dependency can be when I started the month, viewing sugar in the same light as I did alcohol during my dry month. Instead, I began the month thinking I could have a cookie here and there—after all, I knew that kids eat chocolate chip cookies; they serve them in schools and they're not drugs per se. But this rationalization was my undoing: having even a little sweet stuff triggered a vicious cycle of dopamine and dependency, and reward and craving, that makes sugar as addictive as street drugs. My best advice: view sugar like a drug or toxin, not an innocent ingredient, and one that will dramatically affect how you look, feel, and are able to subsist in a matter of minutes.

10. DON'T BE AFRAID TO RESET IF YOU FAIL. Even if you start the month with the best intentions, you may find yourself soon after staring down the empty sleeve of some cookies or at the

bare bottom of an ice-cream pint. If and when this happens, do not beat yourself up. It's difficult to give up the sugar drug, especially if you, like most Americans, have been over-consuming it for years.

But don't let yourself off the hook, either. There are tremen-dous benefits to seeing this challenge to the end, to the best of your ability. You have an opportunity now to try to break free from the cycle of cravings and no control that nobody likes—and that has a deleterious effect on every part of your body, brain, diet, skin, and sleep. Even attempting to take on this challenge gives you the chance to learn which foods in your daily diet contain the most added sugar, and to try to retrain your taste buds so that you can lose even a little dependency on the sweet drug.

Breaking free from sugar is an amazing feeling that can change your life, not just how you look and feel. Don't let one, two, or twenty failures stand in your way of trying to meet that goal. And remember, like I learned, don't be afraid to fail: it will likely teach you more about yourself than a dozen successes.

10

OCTOBER

Stretching

My Story

By this time in the year, I was pretty pleased with my challenge efforts to date. I was continuing to meditate, drink more water, eat less meat, walk anytime I could, and get in regular cardio sessions. I was also still very mindful of my daily phone use and weekly alcohol consumption and was bent on making this month the successful one for my Less Sugar Challenge. And while I didn't do them every morning, push-ups and planks were now ingrained in my weekly routine.

What I realized, though, is that I hadn't done anything that would improve muscle recovery and relaxation, which was increasingly becoming more important as I looked to stay active as I aged. Regardless of how old I was, as a physician, I also knew muscle recovery and relaxation were critical, especially for those who weren't active, since a sedentary lifestyle can lead to more physiological problems than participating in moderate exercise.

That's how I came to settle on stretching as a monthly challenge. The activity was also easy to do anywhere, anytime, with no gym membership or special equipment, and would be beneficial to everyone from elite athletes and weekend warriors to couch potatoes, desk jockeys, and anyone in between. Finally, from a personal perspective, I hadn't religiously stretched since I played competitive sports in high school and figured that, like in challenges past, I could benefit by taking a dose of the antidote I often recommended to patients.

One reason I didn't stretch prior to this month is that I'm naturally very limber and flexible. I can bend over and put my hands flat on the floor and let my outer thighs and knees rest flat on the floor when I sit in a butterfly position. I can even do a split. Yet even though I've never suffered from a lack of flexibility, I know as a doctor that when patients excel in one facet of health or fitness, they often assume they never need to analyze or modify their behavior in that facet. But in medicine, assuming success is never scientific proof of success. Even seemingly healthy behaviors need to be tested to make sure a patient is, in fact, doing everything he or she can to maintain or improve their wellness in this area.

A few years ago, I took a stretching class while staying at Canyon Ranch, a health-minded resort in Lenox, Massachusetts. The class was only thirty minutes, but within that time, we stretched every muscle head to toe, at times using a foam roller or yoga strap to deepen the stretch. I learned a lot during that class, including that there's no correlation between your flexibility and your need to stretch. In other words, you can be naturally flexible and feel loose and limber, but still have muscles, joints, or ligaments that should be stretched.

I also discovered during that class that you don't need to exercise regularly or even work out at all to have sore or stiff muscles. We can get sore from sitting at a desk, standing too long, driving for hours, or doing any routine activity over and over again, like picking up children or heavy grocery bags. Finally, we also get sore from being too inactive. In short, all our bodies need to be stretched.

Even though I didn't stretch regularly, it does feel good when I do. By making it a challenge, I hoped I'd fall in love with the benefits of daily stretching, so much so that I'd make it part of my regular routine going forward. I'm also often sore after the gym, so I was curious to know whether regular stretching would take away some of this discomfort. Although I didn't necessarily mind feeling sore—it meant my workouts were working—I wondered whether feeling fresh would help me exercise harder more often and more effectively. Finally, I have terrible posture, so I hoped by loosening my back, shoulders, and neck, I'd be able to stand up straighter and feel less stiff and hunched.

One thing I knew going into the month was that I wanted a stretching routine that would work my entire body, specifically my neck, shoulders, back, glutes, hamstrings, quads, and ankles, but also take less than five minutes to do. So I created a daily stretching routine that started with head circles, a few in each direction, followed by range-of-motion exercises for the neck, touching my ear to my shoulder, chin to chest, and the lower part of my head to my upper back. I would do arm circles next, followed by a bear-hug stretch in which you grab the back of your shoulders forcibly. Then, I'd stretch my back in all three planes, bending forward and back, to both sides, and twisting in either direction. For my glutes, hips, and hamstrings, I would bend forward and touch the floor, then hold pigeon pose—a yoga exercise to open up the hips—and do a straddle stretch, spreading my legs to form a triangle while leaning forward. I also wanted to use a foam roller, massaging my spine from my upper back to the sacrum, applying pressure to any sore spots and rolling out both glutes, hamstrings, IT bands, and calves. Finally, I'd end with ankle circles.

Before the month began, I did a dry run of my routine, which took no more than three minutes total. I was ready to go.

Week 1
How Daily Stretching Can Overhaul Your Energy

I woke up on October 1, and just like at the start of my push-ups and planks month, I nearly forgot I was doing a Stretching Challenge. It wasn't a busy morning, but stretching had been so far off my radar for so long—and I wasn't nervous or anxious about this challenge, as I had been before the Cardio, Meditation, and even the Less Meat, More Plants Challenges.

As soon as I climbed into the shower, though, the warm water on my muscles made me remember my mission to get more limber and loose. I decided to stretch as soon I got out, when my muscles were already warm and receptive. On my bedroom floor, I finished the routine in just over three minutes, focusing on breathing deep to relax into each stretch and bringing more energy and oxygen into my muscles and limbs. The duration was similar to my initial round of push-ups and planks, but this took much less effort and brought far more enjoyment.

Afterward, I felt invigorated and revitalized, which surprised me since I hadn't done any blood-pumping, heart-racing, or sweat-generating activity. The sensation was oddly satisfying: I was mentally and emotionally calmer, yet physically energized, as if all my muscles were activated and awake, ready to move more smoothly throughout the day.

The next morning, I woke up eager to stretch—I wanted to experience the same sensation I had the day before—completing the routine right after my morning shower again. The third day, I stretched at night, after I got home from work. I didn't forget in the morning, but I was curious how my body would react after a full day on my feet. I was correct to presume a difference: compared to a morning stretch, when my body was fresh, I felt as though I was untangling a wound and knotted rubber band when I stretched at night, working through the tension and stress of the day. And even though it took just three minutes, the routine also helped get me ready for bed, mentally and physically, allowing me to unwind more quickly after being out of the house and working my typical fourteen-hour day.

The first week, I stretched every day but two. On both occasions, I got distracted in the morning, then couldn't find the motivation once I got home at night. I consoled myself with the fact that I did stretch at a SoulCycle class (cardio!) I took on one of my delinquent days. The classes always end with a three-minute stretch on the bike, which the instructor leads. It's optional, and many participants leave, but I always stay because I figure I've paid for the class so I should get everything I can out of it.

I also intentionally doubled the duration of my routine on the weekend, stretching for more than six minutes both days. I assumed this would feel like a chore, but it was actually an indulgent experience, to move through each exercise at a leisurely pace, holding positions longer and accessing a deeper stretch.

At the end of the week, I realized I was enjoying this immensely. I'd never stretched consistently before, and I had no idea how energizing and rewarding it could be. Better still, my posture was also slightly improved: I was standing straighter, my shoulders relaxed and not hunched. Had I known stretching could correct even a tiny percentage of my perpetual slouching, I would have started doing it years ago. Interestingly, I also felt lighter on my feet, as though it was easier to move my muscles because they were less tense and had better blood flow.

The only hurdle, though, was that, unlike the last few months— with the challenges of Less Sugar, More Steps, Hydration, even Mindful Tech—stretching was fairly easy to dismiss. Because it took only three minutes, required no physical exertion, and didn't have as significant health benefits as Cardio, Hydration, More Steps, and other months' challenges had had, the Stretching Challenge was difficult to prioritize. Then again, I was already seeing benefits after just one week. And if it took little time and no effort, why wasn't I prioritizing it?

Week 2
How Stretching Can Improve Your Workouts

I decided to make it part of my daily ritual to stretch after my morning shower—I had learned during the Meditation, Hydration, and Push-ups and Planks Challenges that tying an activity to a part of my morning routine could help make it a new habit. Although I loved the one after-work stretch I did the first week, I didn't seem to be successful at repeating it: I just always felt too drained after I got home to do anything other than fall into bed.

With this in mind, I stretched five mornings during my second week. The two days I missed, I made up in part by taking a Soul-Cycle class and staying for the stretch. While before I had done so only to get the most bang for my buck out of the class, now I was motivated to make sure I stretched in some way every day, wanting to see if I could also learn any new exercises to incorporate into my routine.

At the end of the week, I felt as if the blood flow throughout my entire body had improved. This wasn't a vague concept anymore: my muscles were qualitatively looser and more limber than I could ever remember, which was particularly significant since I hadn't been tight or tense to begin with. But now I felt more agile and nimble, and my posture continued to improve, even over the prior week. I could even feel a difference when I was just walking around . . . And I liked the feeling.

Something amazing also started to happen in the gym in

Week 2: I felt significantly less sore during my workouts. As a result, I noticed I could lift heavier weights and do more reps. This made me chuckle to myself one night when I was leaving the gym after an especially grueling session. I guess these yogis had been right for centuries: stretching is just as important as exercise to your physical and mental health, yet it was so much easier than nearly everything else I undertook in the gym to try to feel and look better.

Week 3
Stretch in the Morning for Improved Posture Throughout the Day

I didn't start the week with a bang—or bend, I should say—missing two consecutive days of stretching right off the bat. The reason was simple: I didn't follow my typical wake-coffee-shower-stretch morning routine. I didn't have to be on *GMA* either morning, which meant I had more time to do other things and less impetus to stretch right away. By the time I realized I hadn't done my three-minute routine, I had to leave for my medical office—the same fate that kept me from doing push-ups and planks months earlier. Throughout the rest of the second day, I began to miss the positive benefits I had now grown accustomed to, especially the feeling of carrying myself with more grace and agility in an upright posture.

But after I returned to my morning stretching, I noticed I wasn't just standing and walking straighter—my posture was also perceptibly better when I was sitting. This was remarkable because I wasn't even trying to keep my shoulders back or spine straight. Bolstered by this, I started to stretch while sitting at my desk in my medical office, doing neck circles, touching my chin to my chest, and crossing one arm at a time in front of my body.

At the end of the week, I felt more energized and limber and even less sore than I had in Week 2. This made sense to me from a musculoskeletal standpoint: instead of only contracting my muscles, which we all do every time we move or exercise, I was lengthening them. I felt like I was finally uncoiling a telephone cord that had been bound for years—my muscles were suddenly free to move in any way I wanted, as they stretched longer and became more elastic, without any knots or adhesive constrictions to slow me down. And it certainly only helped me that I was continuing to drink more water and get in enough aerobic exercise.

When I went to the gym to lift, I continued to be able to include heavier weights and do more reps, and my range of motion was also better using free weights and machines. I could get the lat pulldown bar closer to my chest, for example, touch my chest to the floor with less effort when doing push-ups, and sit back lower in my seat while squatting. I felt stronger, more upright, and more pulled together, to a greater degree than I had during my Push-ups and Planks Challenge.

For someone who had never stretched regularly before and never even thought I needed to, these benefits were encouraging, especially since it was relatively easy and manageable with my schedule. Remind me: Why didn't I start stretching years ago?

Week 4

How One New Easy Habit Led to Big Physical and Mental Changes

By this point, I looked forward to stretching every morning—I never saw it as an obligation or something I had to do for X number of more days. Physically, it felt better, too. While I hadn't minded the muscle intensity or discomfort when I started stretching—I took both to mean I was targeting a tense muscle or ligament—these feelings were almost entirely gone by the last week. My body had grown accustomed to stretching in a positive physical progression, as if I had worked out all the kinks, soreness, and points of tension.

This began to pay off in the bedroom, too. (Not in *that* way!) I started to notice that whenever I crawled into bed at night, I didn't have that heavy ache that usually settled over my body like a sediment whenever I reverted to a horizontal position after standing and sitting all day. Instead, my muscles felt fresh when I lay down, without any soreness or hint of throbbing. And while I had never woken up cramped or stiff per se, I now felt kind of springy when I climbed out of bed in the morning—and the only adjustment I'd made was stretching regularly.

I continued to feel increasingly lighter and more limber throughout the day, while my posture, surprisingly, kept improving. I no longer had to remind myself to keep my shoulders back or suck in my stomach—it was instinctual. I could see the improvement in the gym, too, whenever I caught a glimpse of myself in the mirror. This was considerable since, whenever I work out, I'm usually too sweaty and tired to even try to stand upright. But now here I was, looking ten times straighter than when the month started without even trying. The next morning, I saw myself on *GMA* and had the same reaction: my posture was incredible on the set, where I normally do try to sit up straighter.

Stretching's benefits weren't just physical, either. Knowing that my posture was better and that my body moved more eloquently was a huge confidence boost. It also forced me to step away from my phone and laptop for a few minutes every day, which not only felt great after my recent Mindful Tech Challenge but also seemed like true self-care to me. While the act of stretching in itself was undoubtedly calming, the relaxation lasted nearly the entire day. It was similar to what I felt after a good, deep massage, which would leave my mind and body in a state of zen for hours afterward. Without any physical tension in my muscles, I felt like I had less tension in my life, mentally and emotionally.

At the end of the month, I realized I was silly to ignore stretching just because I was flexible—it was almost like ignoring my sugar intake because I assumed, wrongly as I found out in September, that I didn't have a sweet tooth. Spending just a few minutes a day relaxing my muscles and working on my body's range of motion was having a significant impact on how I carried myself, how I felt about myself, and how I was able to handle stress—I couldn't think of a challenge with a greater return on investment. After all, I probably spent more time waiting for elevators than I did stretching this month.

From a medical perspective, the challenge confirmed what I knew about my patients and had learned during my Less Sugar Challenge: even if you assume you excel in one area of your health and wellness, you can still benefit from analyzing your behavior and seeing if and how you might improve. This was a huge epiphany for me! If I had kept assuming I didn't need to stretch, I would have never realized all these amazing benefits, including improved posture and the ability to work out harder and more effectively, which are two goals I've been chasing down for years.

There was also another lesson for me at the end of the month: don't ignore the health and wellness tweaks that seem easy or nonspecific in theory. Sometimes, the smallest, simplest changes are the ones that can have the most profound effects.

OCTOBER STRETCHING:
The Science Behind Stretching

Most Americans don't stretch, even though it's been shown extensively by research to be immensely beneficial to our overall health. According to the science, stretching is critical to helping muscles stay strong and healthy, regardless of how much or whether you even work out. But the activity, when practiced regularly, can also improve quality of life in some surprising ways. Here's how stretching, even for just a few minutes daily, can overhaul your health.

How and When You Stretch Matters

The science of stretching has progressed immensely since phys-ed class when your gym teacher asked you to touch your toes. This type of stretching is called *static stretching*, or when you assume a position and hold it with your hand, the floor, or the help of a band or partner. By comparison, when you practice *dynamic stretching*, you move your arms, legs, torso, or neck to activate, elongate, and stretch your muscles. Think leg swings, lunges, torso twists, and high knees. There are other types of stretching, too, some of which involve more complicated protocols or aren't recommended by sports medicine doctors.

Today, most experts, including those at the American Council on Exercise, recommend dynamic stretching whenever your muscles are cold to increase blood flow and mobility, and static stretching after a warm-up or workout to relax muscles and promote flexibility. If you don't exercise, practicing both dynamic and static stretching can help bring critical blood flow to undernourished muscles, activate parts of the body not used regularly, increase mobility and range of motion, and help lengthen and relax muscles that are stiff from too much sitting or too little activity.

Stretching Strengthens Muscles and Prevents Injuries

Sitting all day, as most Americans do, is terrible for your body, in part by tightening and weakening muscles, and making it impossible for them to extend fully. Going for a run, hitting the gym, or playing a pickup softball game on the weekend won't necessarily undo the damage, because tight muscles injure easily. Instead, stretching helps keep muscles long and strong, counteracting the deleterious effects of sitting.

While stretching has been fingered as a cause of injury, that's because most people stretch improperly. Static stretching before a workout or whenever your body isn't warmed up can damage muscles, tendons, and ligaments. Dynamic stretching, on the other hand, helps prevent injuries by boosting the flow of blood, oxygen, and nutrients to muscles so your body can move and perform better.

Getting More Limber Can Overhaul Your Posture and Improve Your Appearance

Stretching also prevents injuries by improving posture and helping your body better support your spine and all its moving muscles. But that's not the only reason to try to stand and sit straighter: studies show bad posture is one of the primary causes of low-back pain, which affects most Americans, and can interfere with digestion, cause lasting nerve problems, affect your breathing, and make it easier to fall.

Not standing up straight, as I know, also affects mood and mental outlook. Try it yourself: Do you feel more confident or powerful when you sit and stand up straight, with your shoulders back, your stomach in, and your hips tucked under? Studies show good posture has a significant effect on our confidence and energy levels, reducing stress and negative emotions while making us more productive and alert.

Stretching Can Boost Your Mood More Than Cocktails or Cookies

As it turns out, science shows stretching triggers your brain to release dopamine, that feel-good chemical also created by drugs, alcohol, and sugar. But unlike these unhealthy vices, stretching doesn't cause a commensurate crash or feed a vicious cycle of craving and withdrawal. After all, no one lost her job, ruined a relationship, gained weight, or wrecked her health or life from stretching.

The mood benefits of a good stretch aren't limited to a quick dopamine hit. Studies show regular stretching helps to reduce stress, to relieve anxiety, and even to reduce depression, in a similar way that yoga, meditation, and other mind-body activities can improve our mental and emotional health. Independent of its effects on posture, stretching has also been shown to help increase energy and overall self-esteem.

Foam Rollers Turn Simple Stretching into Self-Massage

Most people don't think of foam rollers when they think of stretching, but that's exactly what these inexpensive, lightweight cylinders are designed for. More precisely, foam rollers let you practice something called self-myofascial release, which is a type of self-massage that helps reduce tension, tightness, and the formation of trigger points, or knots that develop in muscles and tendons.

According to the American Council on Exercise, foam rollers help break up adhesions that form between muscles due to inactivity, poor posture, too much sitting, or repetitive motions like running, cycling, or lifting weights. Left untreated, these adhesions shorten muscles, restricting your ability to move while creating painful knots, or trigger points, between tissues and tendons. The best way to release these trigger points is through massage, whether you hire a therapist or find a few minutes to treat the knot with a foam roller. And obviously, the foam roller is much cheaper than a masseuse!

In addition, using a foam roller regularly has been shown to help lower inflammation, increase blood flow, and trigger feelings of calm and relaxation. Studies also show regular foam rolling can also boost exercise performance over time, helping you work out harder, longer, and stronger.

Stretching Helps Prevent Heart Disease, Diabetes, Cancer, and Other Illnesses

Stretching's benefits reach beyond muscles, ligaments, and tendons. Perhaps one of stretching's most profound effects on overall health is its ability to seem to make arteries more elastic, improving blood flow, preventing stiffening, and reducing the risk of heart disease, according to research. Studies also show stretching is associated with lower blood pressure, LDL cholesterol, and blood sugar, all of which can boost heart health and help lower the risk of other chronic diseases like diabetes and dementia. Stretching may even have an impact on cancer. A 2018 animal study published in *Scientific Reports* shows stretching was associated with the shrinkage of cancerous tumors, which researchers credit to the fact the activity helps improve immune function and reduce inflammation. (Note that I am not suggesting treating cancer exclusively with stretching!)

Research also shows stretching helps people with arthritis or chronic pain better maintain their flexibility and range of motion, curtailing joint pain. If you currently have any type of musculoskeletal pain or injury, stretching can be uncomfortable at first, but this discomfort diminishes when you relax into stretches and disappears entirely when you stretch regularly. Speak with a sports medicine doctor, physical therapist, or chiropractor before undertaking any stretching routine to make sure you don't include any exercises that might aggravate your specific condition.

Stretch During the Day to Sleep Better at Night

If you've read this much about stretching's benefits, it's probably not surprising to learn an activity shown to increase blood flow and boost mood while reducing blood pressure, pain, tension, and stress can also help you sleep better. Specialists say stretching before bed speeds the body's ability to fall asleep while improving your sleep quality throughout the night. At the same time, stretching in the morning can also improve sleep by boosting your energy, mood, and positivity throughout the day, allowing you to better handle the stress that keeps us up at night. Regardless of when you do it, stretching also improves posture while reducing muscle tension and joint pain, reducing the chance you'll be kept up by a bad back, sore muscles, or throbbing knee.

Think of Stretching Like Exercise and Eating Healthy: Results Aren't Overnight

Stretching doesn't work like a superpill, taking away all your back pain or increasing confidence and happiness for days on end. Just like exercise and diet, stretching's benefits happen when you practice regularly and over time. In short, don't give up because you don't feel any differently after a day or two. The longer and more regularly you stretch, the greater results you'll see.

OCTOBER STRETCHING: Your Story

Stretching takes no effort, sweat, or sacrifices and requires only a few minutes daily to produce big results. Despite these advantages, few of us stretch regularly—it's simply not part of the average American's routine. Here are ten ways to change that and make stretching a daily habit capable of overhauling your health and happiness.

1. NEVER STRETCH A COLD MUSCLE. This may seem like stretching 101, but it doesn't stop all the people I see in the gym who assume these awkward positions out of nowhere to stretch

before they work out. The truth is, though, this kind of static stretching, or pushing a muscle into a stationary position before you exercise or even go about your day, increases the risk of pulls and tears and reduces your body's ability to perform well. If you want to warm up before hitting the gym or trails, or before you start the day, do dynamic stretches like walking lunges, leg swings, and neck circles first to bring blood and oxygen into cold muscles.

2. CREATE A COMPREHENSIVE STRETCHING ROUTINE. The best routine starts with dynamic stretches before progressing to static stretches and works the entire body, head to toe, not just those muscles you feel are tight—oftentimes it's the muscles, tendons, and ligaments we don't feel that most need to be stretched since they're pulling on other muscles, creating tightness there. Remember, too, if you stretch the left side, you need to stretch your right and vice versa, regardless of whether you have tightness on both sides. Addressing only one side can create or worsen muscle imbalances and asymmetry.

3. CONSIDER TAKING A CLASS OR GOING ONLINE TO DISCOVER NEW STRETCHES. I learned an incredible amount from taking one thirty-minute class at Canyon Ranch. If you're new to stretching, consider getting an education in new exercises and techniques by taking a class that includes stretching, like yoga, tai chi, or Pilates. No gym membership? Look online for respectable sources like the American Council on Exercise, which offers videos illustrating how to do both dynamic and static stretches.

4. HOLD A STATIC STRETCH, BUT DON'T OVEREXTEND OR BOUNCE. According to the American College of Sports Medicine, you'll get the most bang for your buck by holding a

static stretch for one minute, whether you stay in the same position for sixty consecutive seconds or break it up into three twenty-second intervals. Either way, never hold a stretch that feels painful or reach so far it creates discomfort, both of which can create inflammation and put you at risk of injury. Finally, don't bounce or try to catapult yourself forward past your body's natural range of motion during a static stretch, which can cause injury and muscle soreness.

5. INVEST IN A FOAM ROLLER. The $20 I spent on a foam roller is one of the best investments I've ever made for my muscular health. That's because foam rollers allow you to massage your body whenever you feel a need to, without a pricey trip to a spa or sports therapist. Foam rollers help release muscle tension, tightness, and trigger points in a way even the most comprehensive dynamic and static stretching routine won't be able to accomplish. For all these reasons, I keep my foam roller in my clothes closet, so I'm reminded to roll every time I dress.

6. MAKE STRETCHING A HABIT BY PICKING AND STICKING TO A SPECIFIC TIME. Since stretching is so easy to do, it's also easy to put off, until it's the end of the day and it's too late. In the first week of the month, experiment to find a time in your schedule when you can and will be the most likely to stretch every day. For me, early mornings work best when I'm less likely to be distracted or preoccupied by work or personal matters—it's also when I shower, which provides a natural warm-up for safer, deeper stretching.

    If you work out or go to the gym most days a week, though, you may find it more convenient to stretch after you exercise. If you're not a morning person or struggle to fall asleep, you might find it most beneficial to stretch right before bed. If you opt for an evening stretch, just make sure it's something you can sustain at least five days a week, not only on weekends or nights when you're not out late or distracted by a spouse or child.

7.   TAKE A FASHION BREAK. One reason I recommend stretching first thing in the morning, before bed at night, or after a workout is that you're likely to already be in underwear, pajamas, or exercise clothes—all conducive to a comprehensive stretching routine. Otherwise, you risk a full-body stretch in a suit, pencil skirt, or jeans, all of which won't just be uncomfortable, but also counterproductive. If the only time you can find to regularly stretch during your day is at work, consider keeping a pair of shorts or loose-fitting pants in your office.

8.   THERE'S NOTHING WRONG WITH SOME EXTRA STRETCHING. Stretching feels good, and the more you do it this month, the better you'll feel. I discovered I wanted to stretch in the middle of the day while sitting at my desk—I still stretched most mornings, but these additional bursts were a source of extra energy and relaxation during the day. You may find it easier to incorporate some stretching while standing in a grocery line, waiting for the elevator, or waiting to pick up the kids after school. While you shouldn't rely on spontaneous stretching in lieu of a regular routine, stretching throughout the day will only increase your flexibility, range of motion, muscle strength, energy level, and feel-good mood.

9.   REMEMBER TO BREATHE—AND RELAX YOUR FACE! Whenever we feel uncomfortable, our natural instinct is to hold our breath. But doing so only increases discomfort and anxiety by keeping oxygen from coming into the body when we need it most. For this reason, whenever you stretch, remember to exhale into a position, which will help counter

any discomfort you might feel while allowing you to find a deeper stretch.

Remember, also, not to screw up your face when you stretch. This is a trick I've learned as an ob-gyn. When you tell a woman in labor to relax her face during contractions, she suddenly relaxes her whole body, easing the pain and helping her to give birth more quickly and easily. The same is true when you stretch: relaxing your face will relax your entire body, allowing you to stretch deeper and more comfortably.

10. FIGHT STRETCHING BOREDOM WITH VISUALIZATION. Perhaps the biggest hurdle to making stretching a daily habit is that most of us are easily bored by it. But instead of flipping on the TV or stretching in front of your phone, try to use these precious minutes to totally unplug and allow your mind and body to fully relax. If you find yourself rushing through your routine, try visualization: every time you stretch, think about making each muscle longer and more limber. Studies show practicing this kind of visualization can help you achieve results more quickly and successfully.

11

NOVEMBER

Sleep

My Story

For the last two months, I had challenged myself to improve aspects of my health—my sugar consumption and stretching—in which I mistakenly assumed I was naturally near perfection. Afterward, I discovered new things about myself and ways to improve how I approached both habits that could help overhaul my health and happiness. So for November, excited by the unexpected things I'd discovered, I decided to do the same thing, focusing this month on another aspect in which I assumed I was near perfect: sleep.

I've always been a good sleeper. During college and med school, I could literally put my head on any desk, no matter what was happening around me, and grab a quick snooze, waking up whenever I needed to as if I had a built-in internal time clock. Just ask my good friend and classmate Richard, who would marvel at this ability! When I was on call and working overnight shifts later in my career, I shamed the other doctors by being able to fall asleep anywhere, anytime, almost on demand. I've never had a problem falling asleep or staying there, and I almost never feel tired during the day—if anything, my energy levels are higher than most I know. Finally, I pride myself on a consistent sleep-wake cycle, meaning I get up and go to bed at almost the same time nearly every day—a habit recommended by experts for optimal sleep hygiene.

But life has gotten busier over the last few years, and since I've been at *GMA*, I know my new schedule, with its 5 A.M. wake-up time, has taken a toll on my sleep. Before *GMA*, if I had to guess, I'd say I averaged at least eight hours of sleep per night, unless I was up all night with a patient in labor. Prior to this month's challenge, though, I'd guess I averaged somewhere in the seven-hour range— definitely not bad, but still less than what I was accustomed to. I was curious to know whether trying to get that extra thirty minutes to an hour back would make any difference in my energy, appetite, workouts, or mental acuity. Moreover, I've always seen sleep as one of life's most valuable commodities, and now that my own kids are fully grown, I don't like to compromise sleep for anyone unless it's absolutely imperative to work.

In considering sleep as a monthly mission, I knew the challenge would hit home for tons of viewers and readers. According to the CDC, one in three Americans is clinically sleep deprived, which I see all the time in my practice. I also knew getting more sleep is easier said than done, and when I thought about how to design the challenge, I settled on trying to target at least twenty minutes more sleep per night—everyone is unique, but I thought this would be ideal for me. The more, the better, I figured, but I didn't want to set a goal too greedy or unrealistic to my current schedule. Plus, I assumed I was already at a healthy baseline and really didn't even need more sleep. How wrong I turned out to be.

Just One Night of Poor Sleep Can Affect Your Mood and Energy Levels

The first day of the month was exceedingly busy, with *GMA* in the morning, patients during the day, and dinner with friends at night, when I had two glasses of wine—an amount I hadn't had often since my Dry Challenge (since then I've tried to drink only one serving of alcohol when I go out) and not exactly conducive to healthier sleep habits. But I still managed to get into bed at 9:45 P.M., waking up at 5:15 A.M. the next morning for seven and a half hours of sleep—thirty minutes more than I normally might get.

The next night, a Friday, my boyfriend came for the weekend to celebrate his birthday. We had a wonderful dinner, staying out far later than I normally would despite the fact I had a Saturday *GMA* appearance the next morning. The end result was lots of fun, but little sleep, with only six hours, which left me feeling drained the next day. I did some stretching after *GMA* to try to reenergize my day, then grabbed a forty-five-minute nap, assuming we would be out late that night, too, which we were.

While I didn't have *GMA* Sunday morning, I can hardly ever sleep past 6 A.M.—my internal clock is already set. This meant another night of only six hours of sleep—and a subsequent day of feeling tired, sluggish, and mentally drained. Ironically, this was a great realization: If I felt this much worse after two nights sleeping one hour less than I normally do, how much better would I feel after two nights of sleeping one hour more?

Sunday night, I logged an impressive eight hours, twenty minutes in bed, purposefully going to sleep as early as I could, although my body hardly needed convincing since I was so tired. I know you can never make up for lost sleep, but I woke up feeling wonderfully refreshed the following day.

After the weekend's events, I began to wonder how I could make this month's challenge more effective. Then it dawned on me: Why was I writing down on paper how many hours I slept each night when there was undoubtedly an app to do it for me? I did some online research and settled on a free smartphone app called Sleep Cycle, which tracks total sleep time based on sound and movement while providing interesting stats like total amount of regular sleep compared to deep sleep time. From my More Steps Challenge, I knew using an app could help hold me accountable while making me excited to log successful results.

That night, I switched on the app and put my phone by my bed in its Do Not Disturb mode. The next morning, when I opened the app, I was surprised to see I'd slept seven hours, thirty-seven minutes—I had thought I'd logged no more than seven hours. To date, I'd just been averaging my total sleep time, ballparking when I went to bed and woke up. But now, I had a way to track my sleep more precisely—and I was immensely excited.

The last night of the week, I didn't have any plans, so I decided to take advantage of the low-key evening. I did some evening push-ups and planks along with some stretching to avoid mindlessly scrolling through social media (see how I'm combining three monthly challenges at once there?), then, armed with my new ability to gather specific data, I logged eight hours, twenty-five minutes of sleep, going to bed as intentionally early as I could.

At the end of the week, after three consecutive nights sleeping at least thirty minutes over my average, I was starting to feel better than I had before the month's start. I realized that ending the week with downtime had allowed me to focus on making a conscious effort to sleep more rather than letting it happen by chance. The app also made me eager for the next week to see just how much sleep I could now accurately, precisely, and soundly log.

Figuring Out How Much Sleep You Really Need

For most of the second week, I tried to get into bed as early as I could. I don't like to waste time at night, but like anyone, I can get distracted by certain activities while trying to unwind—even though I've tried to be more careful since my Mindful Tech Challenge, I can still end up online shopping or oftentimes I'll watch *Fauda* on Netflix or FaceTime with my boyfriend or one of my kids at school. But this week, I applied the same discipline I have for getting to the gym to getting to bed. I turned it into a fun challenge to see how many more minutes of sleep I could log by getting into bed before getting sidetracked by time-sucking stuff. Some of these nights, I didn't feel tired, but still forced myself to get into bed—and was still able to fall asleep quickly.

What strengthened my sleep focus this week was that I didn't have any after-work commitments, which was rare, but welcome. I also didn't have any travel, hockey games, or social plans that weekend, which was partly accidental, but once I realized it, I purposely decided not to make any plans so I could focus on sleep.

Three nights that week, I logged fifteen to thirty minutes more sleep than I normally did. The rest of the week, I was at or above the eight-hour mark, with one night at eight hours, thirty minutes, and a remarkable nine hours, nineteen minutes of sleep Saturday night. The morning after this luxurious amount of shut-eye, I didn't feel groggy—just superbly relaxed, as though I was on vacation. I was still continuing to drink more water before bed and was happy to see the increased hydration wasn't making me have to get up to go to the bathroom more than once per night or negatively impacting my total time in bed.

Several factors seemed to point me in the direction of learning the amount of sleep I needed. The days after I slept eight or more hours, I was noticeably more energetic than I had been on my standard diet of seven hours. I also noticed I was less hungry—

woot woot!—and more positive and mentally sharp throughout the day. I even thought my skin had started to look slightly healthier. Reviewing the data on my phone, I could see this was the consistent conclusion: whenever I got eight hours of sleep, I felt better than when I logged seven hours or seven hours, thirty minutes or somewhere in between. If these results kept up through the month, I would have a new challenge: figuring out what I needed to change to ensure I slept eight hours most nights of the week.

For the rest of the month, though, I knew that if I wanted to keep sleeping for eight hours, I had to focus on continuing to go to bed earlier rather than trying to sleep later the next day. With *GMA*, I can't really mess around with my wake-up time: it's usually 5 A.M., or 5:20 A.M. at the latest, although it can be as early as 4:20 A.M. Even if I don't have to be at the studio in the morning, I still instinctually wake up around the same time—a habit I want to keep, too, since I know consistently going to bed and getting up at the same time is key to overall sleep health. Long story short, if I wanted to guarantee myself eight hours of sleep, I needed to be in bed between 9 and 9:30 P.M.

These developments and realizations were all 100 percent positive. Unlike my less-sugar month, there was no struggle here. And it didn't appear as though I'd have to make a massive change to get massive results.

Meanwhile, I had discovered I loved using the app. The technology was holding me accountable for my sleep while adding a scientific element that excited me. Simple to use, the app turned the challenge into an amusing game: knowing my phone was tracking every minute, I wanted to see just how early I could get into bed so I could start the next day off with a feeling of accomplishment when I saw my results. As an unexpected benefit, the app was also preventing me from using my phone at night because it would stop tracking my results if I picked it up to see a text or check email.

Week 3
How to Stress Less So You Can Sleep More

The third week had a rough start. While I thought I'd nailed the solution to sleeping more—I just had to go to bed earlier—I hadn't exactly figured out a strategy for how to accomplish that when I had social plans. My boyfriend was in town again for the weekend, and we had dinner plans—and I hardly wanted to suggest to friends we meet at 5 or 6 P.M. just so I could be home by 8:30 P.M. to go to bed. Instead, we didn't get to sleep until well past 11 P.M. most nights, and while I didn't have *GMA,* I still woke up at 6 A.M., thanks to my internal clock.

But my sleep time still wasn't as disastrous as it had been the first week of the month: I still averaged close to seven hours, thirty minutes of sleep when he was here, with the exception of Sunday, when I logged just under seven hours after going to bed late and having a 4:30 A.M. alarm Monday morning for an unusually early *GMA* obligation.

The night after he left, I slept ten hours, climbing into bed before 8 P.M., which had less to do with the challenge and more to do with the fact I was simply exhausted. But getting that much shut-eye turned out to be a blessing, because the next day, Chloe, Alex, and I left at 10:30 P.M. to drive to Boston to spend Thanksgiving there the following day. We didn't get to Massachusetts until 2:15 in the morning, and when I got into bed at 2:45 A.M., I didn't even bother to turn on the app. Despite the preternaturally late night, I still woke up at 7:45 A.M., five hours later, unable to sleep in much past 6 A.M.

Surrounded by friends and family, I enjoyed myself immensely Thanksgiving Day, but as soon as the sun set, I started to notice my tank was on empty. I was ravenous, and not simply because it was a holiday. I ate more impulsively than I normally would on Thanksgiving, going to bed early and sleeping ten hours, twenty minutes.

Despite hitting my sleep nadir with a five-hour night, I didn't get down about it. I still felt positive about the challenge and that I was above my seven-hour average. Moreover, I knew real life would, at some point or time, get in the way of my sleep schedule, no matter how committed I was to an earlier bedtime. Instead, I vowed that whenever I could control my night, I would be in bed as soon as possible.

While I wasn't too worried about missing a night of sleep here or there, I did now notice that, compared to when the month began, I was less tolerant of subsisting on less sleep. I'd grown used to feeling sharper and livelier, along with being less hungry and cranky, and the effects of a seven-hour sleep—what used to be my normal—were now a negative state I wanted to avoid. This was also partly because, when I didn't sleep enough, the little problems in life felt a lot larger. The month so far had been stressful, as it is for many people around the holidays, but after nights when I got more sleep, the stress felt more manageable. This wasn't because my problems suddenly dissipated or solutions magically manifested. At the end of three weeks, I could recognize the pattern: the more rest I got, the less stress I felt, which helped me prevent problems from turning into full-on catastrophes. While trying to sleep more, I also prioritized continuing to wake up earlier when I could to make sure I could meditate, which I knew was critical to keeping my stress levels in check.

Week 4

How Getting More Sleep Can Help You Lose Weight, Look Younger, and Feel Happier

The last week of the month, I finally cracked the code for how to have a social life *and* get a good night's sleep. It was a busy week between work, social outings, early-morning *GMA* segments, last-minute freelance projects, and weekend hockey games with Chloe. I decided early in the week I could do it all if I was simply strategic about my time, prioritizing getting home earlier to get to bed. The nights I had events or dinners after work, I purposely tried to leave at an appropriate time rather than allowing myself to linger, and soon after I walked in the door, I started preparing for bed, staying away from my phone and doing the little habitual things that let my body and brain know it's time for sleep.

The nights I went straight home after work, I was still busy with *GMA* prep and other projects, but remained conscientious about finishing what I needed to effectively and efficiently so I could go to bed. This didn't require any draconian discipline on my end—instead, it felt like a slap-happy race to beat the clock. While I often wasn't tired when I climbed into bed, I still fell asleep quickly, in part because I'd been training all month for an earlier bedtime.

To finish the month, I logged six consecutive nights of eight hours of sleep. My only seven-hour hiccup happened at the beginning of the week, when I hadn't quite yet mastered the art of leaving an event without lingering.

I felt fantastic. By this, I don't mean I was bouncing off the walls like a five-year-old. Instead, I felt more self-possessed and even-tempered, yet more spirited and mentally sharper—the same sort of results I had seen during my Meditation Challenge. I was more productive, efficient, effective, and—a new adjective for the month—noticeably happier. With more sleep, I felt better about myself and life at large. I also felt more social. While I sometimes view work and social outings as obligations when I'm busy or in a particularly stressful time, despite dealing with both during Week 4, I wanted to go out, see friends and colleagues, and put my best foot forward.

Sleeping more didn't motivate me just to be more social—it also gave me the time, energy, and emotional bandwidth to do things I've wanted to do, like make sure I get in my daily steps, aerobic workouts, and push-ups and planks. Every day in Week 4, I meditated for twenty minutes since I knew my stress levels were high, and I tried to drink more water and eat more plants along with less meat and sugar—all habits I knew would help me feel my best no matter what.

I also experienced a significant drop in my hunger levels—more so than in the weeks prior. This wasn't just placebo effect, either. Earlier in the month, I had begun tracking my diet, logging when and exactly how much I ate on a food app recommended by a friend. Looking back at the data during the fourth week, I was amazed to see how long I was fasting between meals, often going hours without food, also without even realizing it. Normally, if I wake up at 5 A.M., I'm starving by 10:30 A.M. But this week, 10:30 A.M. came and went and I still wasn't thinking about food.

On the last day of the month, Lisa, my makeup artist at *GMA*, paid me a huge compliment: she told me I was glowing. It was something I had noticed, too. Earlier in the week, for the first time in months, I'd decided not to wear foundation into my office, which I habitually do to cover my rosacea. During Week 4, though, I felt I didn't need the makeup because I didn't see the mild irritation and redness that usually spreads across my cheeks. I can't entirely credit this effect to more sleep—after all, association doesn't prove cause—but more sleep was the only thing I'd done differently in the last few weeks.

Using the sleep app helped tremendously, too. By this time, it was habit to turn it on before bed and not touch my phone all night. I felt accountable to my own data and motivated to see positive results. At the end of the month, I did: my average sleep time for the month, or ever since I started using the app midway through the first week, was eight hours, thirteen minutes—a half hour to a full hour more than my norm prior to the challenge. This was a tiny time investment for more energy, less stress, better appetite, healthier skin, and an improved social life. When I thought about how much more productive and efficient I was on an hour's more sleep, spending that sixty extra minutes in bed was no time investment at all.

NOVEMBER SLEEP:
The Science Behind Sleep

Not getting enough sleep can kill you, literally. While that might sound alarmist, what many of us don't realize is that logging less-than-optimal sleep on a regular basis has profound effects on our physical, mental, and emotional health. Even if you think you're doing fine on six hours and don't need a wink more, I can guarantee, as science shows, you're not functioning as well as you might think. Here's why science says we need more sleep than we think.

You Aren't Doing as Well as You Think on Six Hours' Sleep

One of the biggest wellness myths is that some people can sleep six hours or less per night and still function well and be healthy. Instead, every single major medical organization in the country says we need at least seven hours of sleep per night—getting less raises the risk not only of poor mental performance but also of high blood pressure, diabetes, heart disease, obesity, cancer, stroke, and mortality from all causes, according to the CDC. Being chronically sleep deprived can even boost the risk of depression and trigger permanent loss of brain cells.

The only exception to the seven-hour rule is the 1 percent of the population that science has called short-sleepers, or those with a potential genetic variation that allows them to resist the detrimental effects of clinical sleep deprivation; this is most certainly *not* me. Otherwise, 99 percent of us need at least seven hours, if not eight or more, to function optimally. A 2003 study in the journal *Sleep* found that people who slept six hours performed just as poorly on cognitive tests as those who didn't sleep at all for two days straight. Their response time was similar, in fact, to those with a blood alcohol content of 0.1 percent, or legally drunk. What's worse, though, is that the six-hour sleepers all thought they were doing just fine.

Here's another way to think about it: sleep expert Daniel Gartenberg compares six-hour sleepers to fish in a fishbowl. They don't know they're in a bowl until you take them out and set them free in the ocean. Similarly, sleep-deprived people have no idea they're sleep deprived until they start sleeping more.

You Need More Sleep Than You Think

We've all heard that eight hours of sleep is ideal, and studies show people, on average, tend to function best when they get this amount. But how much sleep we each need is largely individual, as research shows our sleep needs are determined in part by our genes, along with lifestyle demands and environment. Some may need nine hours, while others function optimally on seven hours, thirty minutes. The secret is finding your sweet spot when it comes to sleep duration, then sticking with it. But the problem, researchers say, is that most of us overestimate how much sleep we get by at least thirty minutes or more. That means if you assume you're getting seven, you might really be hovering in the low six-hour range.

Getting More Sleep Can Make You Significantly Smarter

Sleeping for eight hours can improve your intelligence, focus, and ability to problem solve. Study after study suggests a good night's sleep has profound effects on different regions of the brain, boosting concentration, reasoning, and the ability to conceive of new ideas and information. Conversely, chronic sleep deprivation can interfere with intelligence, causing the brain to shrink and even causing permanent brain cell loss in gray matter, according to a 2014 study published in the *Journal of Neuroscience*. Studies show people perform up to 60 percent worse on cognitive tests after just five

The Underdiagnosed Sleep Disorder That Can Kill You

If you're overly fatigued or suffer frequent headaches, nighttime sweating, or other symptoms, you may not need a sleep challenge as much as you need to see a doctor. Sleep disorders are common, and while insomnia, restless leg syndrome, and narcolepsy are often easily recognized by patients and their doctors, nearly 80 percent of people with sleep apnea have no idea they have the potentially deadly condition. Women are more likely than men to go undiagnosed.

Symptoms include loud snoring, gasping for air, and not being able to breathe while sleeping. But you don't need to saw logs to have sleep apnea. Because women can't snore as loudly as men due to their smaller airways, female patients, especially those over fifty, when the condition is more common, are more likely to show symptoms like daytime drowsiness, headaches, insomnia, and nighttime sweats. Some of these symptoms are also signs of menopause, which is why it's important to see a doctor who can diagnose the difference. If you have symptoms or are concerned about your sleep habits, see your doctor. Left untreated, sleep apnea can increase the risk of heart attack, stroke, diabetes, and other conditions.

consecutive nights of six hours of sleep or less. What's more, people who don't sleep enough have difficulties learning and remembering information, because the brain encodes what we see and learn every day during the overnight hours. Without enough shut-eye, your brain can't retain information or recall it accurately.

Sleep Is Just as Important as Diet for Weight Loss

How much you sleep is just as important as what you eat when it comes to weight loss, researchers say. Studies show that sleeping less than seven hours can prevent your body from burning fat. One 2010 study from University of Chicago researchers found people lost 55 percent less fat when they got less sleep than those on the same diet who averaged eight hours per night.

Lack of sleep also causes our metabolisms to slow, so much so that scientists even have a term for it: metabolic grogginess. What happens, researchers say, is that after just four nights of reduced shut-eye, your body begins to struggle to process insulin, as its ability to get rid of the fat-storing hormone plunges by as much as 30 percent. What this means is that your body can't clear fat from your bloodstream as quickly, causing you to store more in your cells.

Not sleeping enough impacts your hormones in other ways, too, triggering your body to produce less leptin, the hormone we need to feel full. At the same time, sleep deprivation stimulates the body to pump up production of our hunger hormone ghrelin, along with our stress hormone cortisol, both of which boost appetite levels and food cravings immensely. No matter how much willpower you have, these hormones are hugely influential, causing even the most disciplined and committed among us to lose control around food.

Research from UCLA published in 2017 also shows sleeping six hours or less limits activity in the brain associated with decision making, which can produce an effect on our judgment similar to what happens when we're drunk. Without a fully active frontal lobe, along with increased activity in the brain's reward center, we can't make proper decisions about food or other vices, which is why we're far more likely to cave to any fried food, processed carb, or sugary snack when we haven't had enough sleep.

Not Sleeping Enough Will Wreck Your Skin

Cheat your sleep and it will show up on your face—literally. Being sleep-deprived boosts cortisol, which has an effect on your skin just like it does on your weight. Excess cortisol exacerbates skin inflammation and any related condition, including acne, psoriasis, eczema, and my own issue, rosacea. Too much cortisol also breaks down collagen and hyaluronic acid, both of which help skin stay plump and elastic and (to paraphrase my *GMA* makeup artist) give it its glowing quality. Not enough of either protein can lead to an increase in fine lines and wrinkles.

We also need enough sleep, especially the slow-wave kind, to produce human growth hormone, which is critical to repairing damaged cells of all kinds, including skin cells. Not enough growth hormone also speeds the aging process throughout your body and on the face. Our bodies also use the time we're asleep to rebalance moisture in our skin cells. That's why not sleeping enough can lead to dry skin, along with puffiness and dark under-eye circles that, over time, can become permanent facial fixtures.

Sleep Can Make You Happier and Sexier

Everyone knows a bad night's sleep will make you cranky and grumpy. But sleep's effect on mood goes beyond these surface symptoms of irritability. In fact, a 2017 study from researchers at Oxford Economics found the single biggest factor in living well— more important than money, sex, or even having an extensive support network—was sleep. Getting enough sleep not only increases feelings of elation and positivity, it also boosts self-esteem and limits anger, hostility, and sadness, research shows. When we're well rested, we're also more likely to react appropriately to situations, handle stress well, and find solutions to problems than when we're functioning on low sleep levels.

As I saw firsthand during my Sleep Challenge, we're also more likely to want to be social when we consistently log eight hours. This effect stems in part from increased feelings of positivity, but a 2016 study published in the *Journal of Psychophysiology* also shows getting more sleep makes us more empathetic. Conversely, sleep deprivation prevents people from picking up on social cues from others and can trigger possible inappropriate behavior that we can't recognize in ourselves because we're simply too tired. Yikes!

Sleep deprivation can also take a tremendous toll on romantic relationships, both in and out of the bedroom. For starters, sleep deprivation will kill even the healthiest sex drive, research shows, in part because the body produces the sex hormone testosterone at night. Yet sleep deprivation also drains energy and self-esteem, increasing feelings of tension and hostility, all of which can be borne out in the bedroom.

Study after study also shows couples simply don't get along as well when one or both get less than seven hours of sleep: they're more likely to use negative words, pick fights for no reason, and make impetuous decisions that can interfere with relationship satisfaction. If all this isn't bad enough, sleep deprivation can even make you look less attractive to your partner and others, research shows. A 2017 study published in *Royal Society Open Science Journal* found people rate those who are sleep deprived as less desirable than individuals who get enough shut-eye.

Hormonal Changes Might Mean You Need More Sleep

Estrogen and progesterone help induce sleep, which is why hormonal changes like pregnancy, perimenopause, menopause, and even disruptions in a woman's monthly cycle can cause sleep disturbances. When estrogen and progesterone levels decline during perimenopause or menopause, for example, the hormonal drop can prevent women from falling asleep and cause them to wake up in the middle of the night, triggering hot flashes, especially during the first half of their sleep cycle. Fluctuating hormone levels during pregnancy and postpartum can also cause sleep disturbances, which can increase the risk of postpartum depression.

While these issues are common, you don't have to accept hormonal-related sleep disturbances as part of your lot as a woman. If you suspect hormonal imbalances or changes are causing sleep disturbances, speak with your doctor or ob-gyn. She or he may recommend hormone replacement therapy, along with proven sleep-inducing techniques, like relaxation therapy, paced breathing, and guided imagery. You can also take steps on your own to limit sleep disturbances caused by hormonal changes: exercise on a regular basis; practice meditation, yoga, or other stress-reducing activities; and follow a healthy diet to help limit hormonal imbalances. Either way, the answer to any sleep problem is not long-term or lifelong use of prescription sleeping pills, which just puts a Band-Aid on a bigger problem and will eventually cause more problems than it fixes.

NOVEMBER SLEEP: Your Story

Learning the secrets of more sleep won't just make you successful at this month's challenge—it can also transform your health and happiness. At the same time, sleeping is similar to dieting: there is a ton of advice to be found and many ways to do it well, yet what works for others may not work for you. But there are some universal tips and tricks that can help anyone sleep longer and more soundly. Here are some, along with what I found to be most helpful in making sure you sleep eight hours per night.

1. THINK OF SLEEP AS NONNEGOTIABLE. When work, social life, family, or fun outings suddenly crop up, the first thing to go is often our sleep, as most of us figure we can go to bed later, wake up earlier, or simply miss out on a sound night in order to do what we need or want to do. But this attitude, that sleep is the sliding variable, is why so many Americans

are sleep deprived. Sleep truly has a PR problem! We think of it as a luxury, when in reality, it's a medical necessity! So this month, prioritize sleep by making your bedtime nonnegotiable. If you have to work or want to see friends or spend time with family, cut from another area of your schedule (like your TV time or social media use) to accomplish these demands. Additionally, build in at least thirty minutes of downtime before bed, when you don't do work or use technology and you aren't social, to unwind so that you're ready to sleep as soon as you crawl into bed.

2.   CREATE A REGULAR SLEEP SCHEDULE. Going to bed and waking up at the same time every day is one of the most effective ways to establish a healthy sleep routine. A habitual bed pattern will set your body for sleep similar to how meals train your body to eat: if you have dinner around 7 P.M. every night, for example, you know you'll be hungry at this hour nearly every evening. Likewise, a consistent sleep-wake cycle tunes your body's circadian rhythm to these hours, helping you fall asleep faster, wake up more easily, and avoid middle-of-the-night disruptions. Establishing a consistent sleep schedule during the workweek is usually easy—the key is to go to bed and wake up at the same time over the weekends. If you end up staying out late, sleep experts say it's better to wake up at the same time the next day and nap midday than it is to sleep in late on a weekend morning.

3.   REDESIGN YOUR SLEEP ENVIRONMENT. I didn't realize how critical sleep environment is to actual sleeping until later in life. After years of reading the recommendations on how our bedrooms should be dark, cool, and quiet, I finally put up blackout drapes in my bedroom just recently and now always make sure to lower my thermostat into the 60s (studies show anywhere between 60 and 67 degrees Fahrenheit is optimal

for inducing zzz's). Both tweaks have made a big difference in my sleep quality, which is why I suggest anyone interested in prioritizing their sleep make these changes, too.

While I don't have a noise problem at home, if you can't prevent sounds from other rooms, nearby neighbors, or busy outside streets, or you travel frequently, consider running a source of white noise, like a box fan, noise machine, or white noise app on your phone. Studies show white noise masks disruptions in audible frequencies that keep us from falling asleep and staying there.

4. RETHINK WHOM YOU DO AND DON'T SLEEP WITH. Many studies show we don't sleep well when someone else is in our bed, especially if that person snores loudly. If your partner or spouse is keeping you up at night, encourage him or her to see a doctor for any snoring issues, then consider sleeping in separate rooms. Known as a "sleep divorce," or when couples sleep in separate bedrooms, 25 percent of all married Americans do this and report more quality sleep as a result. At the same time, some research shows that women can sleep more soundly when they share a bed with someone they love or who gives them feelings of comfort and security. Another recent study found women sleep more soundly with their dogs than they do with their human partners, who are more likely to disturb them in the middle of the night. I know that whenever my nine-pound Mason shares my bed, he curls up like a little cinnamon roll next to me and I sleep amazingly.

5. ESTABLISH A BEDTIME ROUTINE. Doing the same things every night before you go to bed will give you a bedtime routine that prepares your body physically and mentally for sleep. This way, your body and brain know that when you shut off the lights, wash your face, brush your teeth, light a

candle, and then finally climb into bed to read your favorite book, in that order, it's time to sleep. For optimal shut-eye, avoid eating or drinking large amounts of food or liquid before bed, both of which can interfere with sleep, and be sure to avoid caffeine, alcohol, or late-night exercise, all of which can interfere with rest.

6. USE AN APP. Using an app to track my sleep was a game changer for me this month. The app not only helped me accurately log my sleep, it also held me accountable to the challenge, motivated me to work harder, and added a sense of competitive fun to the month. With the app, I wanted to get into bed as soon as possible so I could see positive results the next day—and I was encouraged to keep going whenever I did.

   An app can also be useful in providing an accurate snapshot of your current sleep habits: according to experts at the University of California–Berkeley and elsewhere, most Americans overestimate how much sleep they get. Many sleep apps are free and offer other benefits as well, like guided meditations to help you sleep and even bedtime stories scientifically shown to induce shut-eye in adults. Whatever you choose, be sure to set your phone on Do Not Disturb at night if your app doesn't automatically do it for you, so you won't be awakened by pings, dings, and chirps.

7. ADOPT A NO-GUILT MIND-SET. No one is going to have a heart attack if you choose to go to bed and there are still dishes in your sink, unanswered emails on your computer, or other chores on your to-do list. While taking care of stressful tasks and preparing for the next morning in advance can help you go to sleep with a clear mind, on many nights you simply won't be able to do everything you want to before you go to bed. And that's okay. Prioritizing sleep is more important

to your health and wellness than even the cleanest kitchen. Also remember that, with a good night's sleep, you'll be more productive and efficient the next day, making all those little tasks so much easier to accomplish.

8. CONTROL WHAT YOU CAN, WHEN YOU CAN. No matter how hard you try, you won't be able to control exactly when you go to bed every single night of the week for the rest of your life. Sick kids, sudden work demands, family emergencies, and special occasions like holiday travel can all interfere with our sleep routines, which is normal. But instead of stressing out about a night or two of missed sleep, try to accept it, do what you can to sleep well during those situations, and then vow to continue prioritizing your sleep when you regain control of your schedule. Otherwise, if you shortchange your sleep on the nights you can control your bedtime and then the unexpected happens, you will fall into a sleep rut that can take days or even weeks to recover from.

9. DITCH THE NONNATURAL SLEEP AIDS. As a physician, the only time I recommend prescription or over-the-counter sleep aids is for short-term use when patients are traveling or facing a period of extreme stress. Otherwise, these drugs impede quality sleep by leaving you sedated but not well rested while interfering with your ability to fall asleep naturally over time. If you have difficulties sleeping, speak with your physician about other ways to address the problem. You can also consider natural alternatives like supplemental melatonin; tea with chamomile or lavender; or supplements that contain valerian root, magnesium, and/or glycine, all of which research shows to induce sleepiness.

10. NOT TIRED? TRY DAYTIME EXERCISE, PRODUCTIVITY, AND SUNLIGHT. If you have trouble falling asleep, you might not

suffer from a sleep disorder as much as you simply aren't expending enough energy or effort during the day. Studies show that exercise is one of nature's most effective sleep aids—if you aren't working out now, add morning or afternoon exercise sessions before you treat your sleep difficulties with anything else.

Another factor that can prevent nighttime sleepiness is not feeling useful or productive during the day. To remedy this, try taking on more responsibilities at work, commit to a new project or class, pursue a hobby, or make more plans with friends or family. Not seeing the daytime sun can also prevent nighttime sleepiness, so be sure to get outside every day, preferably first thing in the morning to help reset your body's internal clock.

12

DECEMBER

Laughter

My Story

For almost one full year, I'd undertaken mostly serious challenges, designed to hard-target improvements in my health and
overall life. Some were difficult to do (I'm looking at you, less sugar
September) and many were high stakes, like avoiding alcohol to cut
breast cancer risk, drinking more water to prevent kidney stones,
and doing more aerobic exercise to slash my incidence of just about
every chronic disease. While I was immensely pleased with what
I'd accomplished in the preceding months, I knew there was something missing, an important aspect of my overall health and wellness picture that I had yet to access.

My challenges to date had mirrored my personality. I'm extremely
driven and like to target quantifiable goals—aims that have statistics
I can apply or derive. I'm not proud of it, but I'm not someone who
works hard, plays hard—I definitely work hard, but I play very little.

For example, for all my four years in college, I bartended three nights a week at one of the hottest places in New York City. And while everyone else my age was letting loose and having fun in an environment designed solely for enjoyment, I was working, making money, and taking it all very seriously.

Fast-forward from college to nearly midlife, and I still don't often do fun for fun's sake. As a doctor and a scientist, I like to quantify my behavior, and it's nearly impossible to quantify amusement like you can an hour-long workout or seeing twenty patients per day in my medical office.

It's not just my personality: my chosen professions, by their nature, are also quite serious. As a doctor, there's little room for silliness or merrymaking at work. When I see patients or look over test results, I need to be 120 percent focused—people's lives are at stake. The same is true as a medical correspondent on *GMA*: millions of people are listening to me give them health advice, so I need to make sure I get nearly every word right.

That said, while I'm a serious person and take what I do seriously, I try not to take myself seriously. I think it's critical to be able to laugh at yourself. Without that ability, how could you handle the mistakes you might make, hardships that arise for no reason, and critical and trivial misfortunes alike that befall everyone? Plus, if you can't count on yourself as a source of entertainment, who *can* you count on?

Over the last few years, I've become more accepting of my mistakes and misfortunes and, consequently, my own flaws and vulnerability. After my ex-husband died by suicide, I realized there was no such thing as a perfect life, only a real life. Tragedy made me want to embrace my real life and who I really am, each and every flawed part.

Today, I tell my children and my patients that life is too short not to be able to learn to accept yourself for who you are. If you want to truly love yourself—and be able to love those around you—you have to embrace your mistakes and flaws as much as you do your strengths and successes. I like to set the bar high for myself every day, but I believe you can't be truly happy and healthy if you're not able to forgive yourself and others—and if others can't forgive you, well, then, they don't deserve to have you in their lives. Otherwise, obsessing over your mistakes and weaknesses—and those you see in others—will eventually eat you up, taking a big toll on physical, mental, and emotional health.

While I've learned to laugh at myself, I haven't been so successful at finding ways to lighten and loosen up. As a result, I'm almost never silly. That might not sound like a big deal, but to me, it means I've lost that precious childlike ability to find joy in all the little things in life. And to me, that is a big deal—and something I want desperately to change.

So for the month of December, I decided to make it my mission to laugh more and rediscover that innate childlike glee we're all born with. While there are many ways to unlock more levity in your life—find a funny YouTube channel you like, spend more time with family and friends who make you laugh, watch comedy shows or sitcoms—I chose a very particular path to silliness that I found, of all places, in my closet. This is not about what you need or should do to bring laughter in your life, but by sharing my specific story, I hope it will help you realize more ways to discover the levity that can make us all healthier and happier.

My daughter, Chloe, has been a tomboy her whole life. When she was young, she preferred playing ice hockey to playing with dolls and had no interest in makeup, dresses, or the other things that often delight little girls. For these reasons, it wasn't entirely surprising when, at age four, she couldn't have cared less about a sparkly plastic princess tiara she got as a favor from someone's birthday party. What was surprising, though, was how that tiny child's crown ended up in my closet—to this day, I have no idea.

When I first discovered the mysterious tiara inside my closet, I decided it was a sign—and one I needed to act upon. From that day forward, I started putting the crown on whenever I wanted to amuse my children, sometimes even meeting their friends wearing the silly thing. This made me laugh out loud: here I was, an adult woman, greeting kids while wearing a cheap, bejeweled toy tiara for no apparent reason other than I was the queen of my own apartment whom the children had to say hi to as they entered my kingdom. My own children also found it funny, joking with their friends that they had two choices: they could either call me "Jen" or "Queen Jen," as Dr. Ashton was out of the question.

Even though my kids are now grown and away at school, the crown has remained in my closet for the last fifteen years—never lost, never broken, but always there among my television dresses, designer shoes, blue jeans, workout clothes, medical scrubs, and all the other very adult, very serious things inside. When I see the tiara there, it makes me smile. I still put it on several times a year, usually when my kids are home or sometimes when FaceTiming with a close friend or my boyfriend.

When I started thinking about how to design a monthlong challenge around laughter, the tiara instantly came to mind. I decided I could wear it just a few minutes every day, at different times and under different circumstances, and try to make myself and others laugh. Let the silliness begin.

Week 1
The Five-Minute Way to Feel Happy All Day

The first few days of the month were immensely busy, so much so that I forgot entirely about the challenge. How could this happen? I'd been looking forward to a lighthearted challenge all year, and it was the easiest one to date—no planks, aerobic exercise, disciplining myself to drink or not drink something, eat or not eat a certain food. Was I really so high-strung and preoccupied that I couldn't take five minutes to put this sucker on my head and laugh? *God,* I thought, *I need some silliness now more than ever.*

On the fourth day, I threw the tiara in my purse before heading out to *GMA*. Once I get to the studio, I usually have about thirty minutes in makeup before I have to get my hair done. So while sitting in the makeup room, I put the tiara on my head while chatting with one of the producers. I had already told her and the other producers about the challenge so they wouldn't be shocked—and this particular producer also has two young children, so nothing seems to faze her. In fact, she was all business as usual while I wore the tiara, which made me chuckle just to think about the image we were projecting, having a very serious conversation while I had the toy tiara on my head.

As I talked with the producer, former White House communications director and ABC and *GMA* anchor George Stephanopoulos walked by and glanced into the room where we were chatting. Despite the fact I had a tiara on my head, George gave me his typical serious and focused "Good morning" nod, without even doing a double take. I just started laughing out loud, only imagining what was going through George's head when, just minutes before air, he had seen the trusted medical correspondent wearing a tiara. As I took it off, I thought, *Wow, this thing really works: I'm laughing.* George and I have still never spoken about the incident, but I have to assume it caused him to chuckle, too—or, at the very least, wonder exactly what was going on with one of his colleagues.

The next day, I wore the crown while going over labs in my medical office. No one saw me except for my staff, who got a kick out of seeing me in my white doctor's coat adorned with this dazzling tiara. I even kept the crown on while telephoning patients to go over their blood test results. This had an amazing effect, reducing significantly the inherent stress I feel when making these calls. While I would never wear a tiara or any other silly item in front of patients—I would never want to diminish the gravity of their health concerns—simply having the thing on helped offset all the concern and solemnity I often feel at work.

The last two days of the week, I wore the tiara around my apartment while FaceTiming with Chloe and my boyfriend. Neither of them was particularly shocked—they'd seen the crown before—but I started laughing. I didn't need to wear it a long time, nor did I necessarily want to, which I felt might be inconsiderate to whomever I was talking with. But just having the crown on my head for a few minutes made me feel lighter, as though I was getting a quick break from the high-stakes seriousness of life.

At the end of the week, I couldn't believe what the crown was doing: just wearing it for five or ten minutes made me feel so much lighter and more buoyant for the rest of the day. This wasn't because those around me would fall down in hysteria when they saw me in the tiara, either. While my colleagues and kids got a kick out of the crown, the joy I experienced was due to my own glee in having a $1 toy tiara on my head.

Why was a cheap crown making me so happy? What the tiara provided, I realized, was an instantaneous break from the grind and gravity of life. Think about it: most of our days are spent working or worrying about money or checking off chores, trying to improve ourselves and our relationships while striving to behave well and perform our best. Altogether, this makes our lives into something like a serious sandwich: you're continually pressed in the middle between what you have to do and what you know you should do. But with the tiara on my head, I was able to pull back the metaphorical bread and move around a little bit on the inside. When I wore the crown, I wasn't thinking about what I had to do or what I should do—instead, I could ignore for a moment what was expected or even appropriate and dial into just enjoying myself. When I had the crown on my head, the stress poured out and some happiness rushed in.

As the week ended, I also started to think about where else I could wear the crown. Could I wear it in public? But what if someone recognized me and assumed I'd had a psychotic break? I decided

I could wear it in the car while driving to my office in New Jersey or even to one of my daughter's hockey games, although the thought made me slightly uncomfortable.

Finding Ways to Feel Joy No Matter Where You Are or What You're Doing

For Week 2, I decided to see what happened if I took the tiara out of my closet and kept it somewhere in open view, where I'd see it every time I walked in and out of my apartment. My kitchen island seemed like the most visible place, so I left it there, hoping the high-traffic spot would encourage me to wear it more. The trick worked: not only did I pick it up more often this week, the mere sight of the tiny, sparkling tiara among my kitchen appliances also made me smile every time I walked by.

To start the week, I wore the crown at five one morning while getting ready for *GMA*. Rushing around making coffee and getting dressed, I caught a reflection of myself in one of my apartment windows, and I started to laugh out loud: here I was, a grown woman, wearing a tiara in the predawn hours as I prepared for my very serious job as a national network medical correspondent. This caused me to practically double over in laughter, which I don't think I've ever done so early in the morning. The crown added just the shot of levity I needed, and when I walked into *GMA* that morning, I felt like I had a secret. I wanted to whisper to my coworkers, *If you could have seen me a half hour ago, you would have peed your pants!* For the next few hours, I had an extra zing in my step, as I kept thinking about my morning.

The following day, I finally did it and wore the tiara in public—or semipublic, I should say. I put the tiara on while driving to my office in New Jersey. As soon as I got behind the wheel, I started chuckling to myself, giddy in anticipation of someone doing a double take after getting a glimpse of a well-coiffed blonde driving a sedan and wearing a cheap child's tiara. But surprisingly, no one seemed to notice. Were people really so programmed, preoccupied, or matter-of-fact? The realization made me chuckle even more, as I thought that I could really do whatever I wanted while driving with the tiara and no one would notice.

The next day, I didn't wear the tiara until the evening, when I was brushing my teeth and getting ready for bed. I was also wearing my usual cuddly winter sleepwear—plaid flannel pajamas—and when I saw myself in the mirror with the bejeweled tiara on, too, I looked hilarious. If you saw me only from the neck up, you would have sworn I had some sexy nightgown on. Instead, I was dressed like I was about to appear in an L.L.Bean ad, except that I was wearing a child's crown.

Later that week, I put the tiara on to walk my dog, Mason. This was not as risqué as it sounds: I was walking him on a private outdoor terrace, where no one could see me. But the fact that I was wearing the crown while doing such an ordinary, everyday task made me smile.

That weekend, I wore the tiara around my apartment, both Saturday and Sunday. By now, I already knew how I was going to react to having the crown on my head—I was almost guaranteed to laugh out loud. But that weekend, I started to wonder how strangers would react and how that would make me feel—that is, if I ever got up the gumption to wear it in public other than within the relative anonymity of my car. The idea of donning the tiara on the streets of New York City made me a little self-conscious—I wasn't sure I had the guts. What if someone recognized me?

When I talked to Chloe about my concerns going public, she told me if it was her challenge, she'd wear the tiara everywhere—to the gym, coffee shop, her classes, even just walking down the street. I suddenly felt as if I was in a Dr. Seuss book: Would I wear it on a train? In the rain? In a box? With a fox? Even thinking about the crown was now amusing me.

I also realized that wearing the tiara, even for just minutes, could lift my mood immediately. At the very least, seeing it in my kitchen would make me smile. Yet I had only worn the tiara when I was in a neutral or positive state. Would it work just as well when I was upset or superstressed? Could I actually use the tiara to help relieve anxious or terrible times? Maybe I should carry the tiara with me everywhere, like I do my exercise resistance bands—in my purse, in my car, at the office, when I travel—so that I'd have a quick way to tap into some joy no matter where I was, similar to how I could get in a workout with the bands anytime I wanted.

A friend once gave me a shirt that read, KEEP CALM AND LET JENNIFER HANDLE IT, with a picture of a crown below the saying. There are lots of images that could have conveyed that same sense of inner strength—a superwoman cape, a spear, a shield, or a pair of clasped hands. But I was beginning to understand that the image of a crown resonates with me because it's so entirely antithetical to who I am. Similar to my daughter, I'm not a girly girl who likes sparkly things, fancy dresses, or princesslike accoutrements that would come with wearing a crown. I prefer jeans and leggings, with my hair pulled back in a ponytail and no makeup on my face except when I'm on TV. Topping this look with a crown was such a comical contradiction, but not necessarily one that wasn't true, since I often feel like I do and can take care of everything.

Week 3
How to Learn to Be Your Own Best Friend

Week 3 in December was insanely busy, like most days are right around the holidays. Between patients, *GMA*, travel plans, and other holiday madness, there wasn't any time to relax, but having the tiara on my kitchen island helped remind me what the season is all about. It also turned down my stress levels every time I saw it there.

Since the crown was always there, I started wearing it more around my apartment, putting it on two mornings that week while making coffee. Even though I had already done the tiara morning routine before, I still found the circumstance just as hilarious. I began to wonder whether I should start every day with the tiara since it was clearly capable of improving my mood immensely. And all I had to do was plop the silly thing on my head for five minutes.

I also wore the tiara twice that week at night, both times while prepping for *GMA* segments. This was a different experience altogether, the crown having a surprisingly calming effect in the evenings, instantly cutting the stress of a hectic day with a pop of pure pleasure. I liked ending the day this way, on a lighthearted and positive note, and I began to wonder whether I should also wear the tiara every night, just to undo the anxiety that inevitably develops during any workday.

That weekend, I traveled to Hawaii for the holiday break—and, of course, I had to bring the tiara. I even wore the crown in the cab to the airport, the whole time feeling like Carrie from *Sex in the City,* laughing to myself while New York City whirled by me. No one saw me other than my kids and the taxi driver, who oddly didn't give me one strange look. But I didn't mind—I was now more interested in enjoying myself than eliciting a chuckle from others.

In fact, I had been mostly laughing by myself this month, I realized, which was hardly typical. Usually, we don't laugh in isolation—we almost always laugh around others or because of others, whether that's with friends or while reading a funny book or watching a comedy show or movie. Think about all the times you've doubled over in laughter, and I bet you were either with someone or a group of friends or you were at a movie or show.

During my Laughter Challenge, though, I was laughing by myself, at myself—in other words, by my own volition. Sometimes it was just a small giggle; other times, it was nearly a laugh-out-loud hysteria. Either way, I realized I was becoming my own best friend, capable of picking myself up and making me laugh whenever I wanted or needed to. Even just thinking about the tiara now could cause me to chuckle. All in all, this meant I had laughed more on my own this month than I had cumulatively in the last decade.

By the end of the week, I still wondered whether I would ever wear the tiara in public. I came close once, grabbing it on my way to an ABC meeting. In the end, I realized I wasn't ready, even though I desperately wanted to be—I had once seen a runner in the New York City marathon wearing a shark costume and it still makes me laugh to this day. But I also wanted to make sure, if I did wear the tiara in public, I did it on my terms, within my comfort level.

Week 4

What Happens When You Start Seeing the World Through a Child's Eyes

I finished the year with one glorious week in Hawaii with my children. This had an interesting effect on the month's challenge: while I wore the tiara in the hotel room most days of the week, it didn't trigger the same deep belly laughs it did when I donned it at home in one of the world's busiest cities while engaged in my superserious jobs.

In Hawaii, things were so easy-breezy that I didn't need the comic relief the crown provided. What's more, I already felt like a queen in Hawaii, like I was walking on air in paradise—when I put on the tiara, it only reinforced those feelings of queenliness rather than working to contrast with my life in New York City as a medical doctor, television correspondent, and parent. In other words, while on vacation in Hawaii, the tiara seemed like an appropriate headpiece rather than a silly aberration.

This only reinforced how valuable the crown was to me in real life. If this cheap child's tiara was natural on vacation, yet comical in the city, then I needed to wear it more often when home to give my life there the humor and amusement it obviously needed.

Later that week, I made a headband out of Hawaiian orchids in a class offered by the hotel. When I placed this exquisite piece on my head, I immediately thought of the plastic tiara waiting upstairs in my room. What a difference there was between the two! With my new orchid crown, I felt like an authentic island queen; with my sparkling plastic tiara, I felt like a playful princess who had a hilarious secret. Both pieces had their place and purpose, and both, I realized, gave a valuable sensation of self-love and comfort that everyone, me included, could benefit from.

Throughout the week, I kept wondering if I'd finally get the guts to wear the crown in public. Here I was, on vacation in an exotic locale with my kids, who'd both encouraged me to wear the tiara out. But I just wasn't able to do it. I was learning something about myself and my own personal boundaries—a realization I would have never expected from this challenge. But I was happy for the opportunity to better understand my own comfort levels.

Forgoing the crown in public certainly didn't diminish any of its benefits. To that end, I realized in the last week that I was laughing more in general than I had ever before—not just when the tiara was on but on all occasions and at all things. I was even alone with my children in Hawaii, not around my peers with whom I could enjoy adult humor. But the crown had opened me up to laughing and enjoying myself more. Laughing, like any other behavior, is partially conditioned, meaning the more you can do it, the more you will do it.

Wearing the tiara had also done something else quite incredible: it made me be in the moment. In Hawaii, I realized I was more engaged in what I was doing when I was doing it than I'd almost ever been before. Putting a toy tiara on my head regularly for four weeks had forced me to step out of my adult world and stop thinking about what I needed to do next, which segments I should prepare for, which patients or personal issues needed my attention, which chores I had to check off my ever-building mental list. With the crown on, though, all I could think about was the silly thing on my head and what I could or would do while wearing it. Being engaged with the tiara on a near-daily basis now carried over into my regular life, putting me more in the moment even when I wasn't wearing the crown.

Perhaps one of the biggest realizations of the week—and the month—came while I was horseback riding in Hawaii. On the ride, I started chatting with the wrangler about Disney World, as Disney is also the parent company of ABC News. The wrangler had never been and I'd only visited for the first time as an adult. On that inaugural trip, I told him, I realized that Disney World was better suited to adults than kids: children don't need any help finding the joy and laughter in life that Disney celebrates—most kids can find both right at home, building a simple blanket fort, playing in a backyard treehouse, or visiting a local playground. But as adults, we lose that childish ability to find amusement and laughter in almost everything, which is why a trip to Disney can be crucial to helping grown-up kids rediscover the joy inside all of us.

As I was telling the wrangler this, it dawned on me that the crown had done the same thing for me that Disney did all those years ago: wearing the tiara had helped me see things as a child, opening my eyes to more joy and laughter everywhere I looked. While I had never expected this challenge to have such an immense effect, I realized this was one of the most valuable lessons I'd learned all year. Without joy and laughter, how could anyone be happy—or healthy? And what would being healthy even mean if you couldn't properly experience all the life and vitality these challenges work so hard to preserve?

DECEMBER LAUGHTER:
The Science Behind Learning to Laugh More

You've heard the maxim many times before: Laughter is the best medicine. Turns out, the saying is based largely in science. The idea that humor can help prevent and even help treat illness and disease has been studied extensively by the medical community since the 1960s. Since then researchers have discovered just how beneficial a good guffaw can be to our overall physical, mental, and emotional health. While it may not surprise you that laughter can help slash stress, just how much it reduces anxiety and tension may amaze you, along with the other incredible benefits of learning to laugh more.

Laughter Is One of the Fastest and Most Effective Ways to Fight Stress

Humor can make you feel instantly happy and allow you to temporarily forget about all your work, financial woes, and personal problems for a quick second. But the power of mirth and merriment goes beyond just temporary stress relief. Studies show laughter lowers levels of adrenaline and the stress hormone cortisol that has been linked to nearly every health condition, including weight gain, skin aging, diabetes, Alzheimer's, cancer, and heart disease. Laughter can slash stress so much, in fact, that even anticipating a good guffaw has been shown to cut cortisol, according to studies.

Laughter doesn't just stop the bad stuff—it also stimulates your body to make more good chemicals, including endorphins, the same hormones triggered by exercise that help you feel more serene after a good sweat session. Additionally, humor stimulates the brain to make more dopamine, the powerful pleasure chemical also boosted by sugar, alcohol, drugs, and other perceived stress relievers that carry detrimental effects that laughter doesn't.

When we laugh, we also give our body a good physical release from stress, as merriment helps to relax muscles, lower blood pressure, and increase oxygen uptake. For these reasons, research shows humor can reduce anxiety levels even more than exercise, according to a 2003 study among college students published in the *Journal of Leisure Research*.

Laugh More to Feel Less Pain and Heal Faster

Comedy is one of the world's oldest ways to distract people from feeling pain—it's why some doctors use humor on patients during surgery before the onset of anesthesia. But it turns out, there's science behind the outdated practice: the endorphin rush you get from laughter and exercise also helps to reduce pain in a powerful way. A 1996 study published in the *Journal of Applied Social Psychology* found that hospital patients who watch funny movies need fewer prescription pain drugs than those who watch other types of TV. Similarly, a 2011 study published in the *Proceedings of the Royal Society* discovered people could withstand the discomfort of ice-cold water longer when they were laughing than when they weren't—their pain tolerance also lasted twenty minutes longer after their humor session subsided. Even the Cancer Treatment Centers of America recommends laughter therapy as a potent palliative for patients suffering intense pain due to the chronic disease.

Laughing Burns Calories, Tones Abdominal Muscles, and Makes You Fitter

---

Think of laughter like a quick aerobic workout, capable of helping your body burn calories, tone its abdominal muscles, increase blood and oxygen flow, lower blood pressure and LDL cholesterol, and even boost overall cardiovascular strength, according to research. According to researchers at Stanford University, laughing a hundred times in one day is the equivalent of a ten-minute aerobic exercise for your body and brain. No, you can't use a comedy show in lieu of a trip to the gym—cardio exercise still has its unique and very impressive benefits—but adding more humor to your daily routine can help you stay fit and lean. And while laughter's metabolic burn won't undo the effect of eating a whole plate of Christmas cookies, you'll still torch up to fifty calories in ten minutes of giggles and guffaws.

Laughter Will Help You Live a Longer and Healthier Life

Research shows laughter has a very laudable effect on the immune system, boosting immune cell activity and the antibodies that help fight infection. In particular, research shows comedy can increase the body's production of T cells—the immune system's most critical disease-fighting cells that target pathogens of all types—and natural killer cells, which attack viruses and tumor cells. Studies have also found that mirth can cause your body to make more immunoglobulin A, an antibody that helps ward off upper-respiratory issues. Additionally, humor's stress-busting, mood-boosting properties do double time for our immune system, fighting off the anxiety, tension, anger, depression, and the overall unhappiness that have been shown to help lead to illness and disease.

Use Laughter Like Therapy to Release Blocked Emotions and Lift Mood

You probably already know humor can make you happy—at least temporarily—but laughter's ability to morph your mood is stronger than momentary merriment. Study after study shows that laughing regularly not only tempers overall anxiety, anger, sadness, and other negative emotions, it also boosts feelings of self-esteem and confidence, social connectiveness with others, and general enjoyment of life that extend beyond the few seconds it takes to get in a good chuckle. In fact, experts at the Mayo Clinic say laughter is so effective in lifting mood that it can be used to help prevent and even help treat depression.

That's not all: perhaps one of the most interesting ways in which laughter can improve psychological health is by helping us release blocked emotions. When we laugh, our inhibitions are temporarily lowered, allowing suppressed emotions to surface—explaining why some people may even feel grief or sadness after a good laugh.

Laughter Makes You More Likable, Successful, and Attractive to Others

Learning to laugh more isn't just good for your health—it can also improve your professional, interpersonal, and romantic lives. When you make someone laugh or you chuckle at another's joke, it creates a shared bond, establishing a sense of understanding and togetherness with that person or group of people. Research also shows we like people more who make us laugh or, conversely, who laugh at our jokes.

For these reasons, humor not only makes you more likable, it can also improve your professional relationships with managers, employees, customers, and potential clients. Laughter has been found to be an effective icebreaker and networking tool, and studies show that humor increases professional trust, productivity, creativity, and team morale among employees.

Laughter can even make you more attractive to others—physically and mentally. Studies show men and women find strangers who laugh or who make them laugh more attractive than those who don't have a strong sense of humor. Psychologists also say laughter can help couples better solve relationship problems and can lead to more successful, longer-lasting relationships and marriages.

Laughing Improves Memory and Makes You Smarter

You may not think that something as simple as a good giggle can boost brain function, but that's the surprising conclusion from several interesting studies. One 2014 study from researchers at Loma Linda University in particular found that humor improves memory recall, along with learning and sight recognition, in part by decreasing cortisol, which can damage brain cells. A 2010 study from researchers at the University of Western Ontario discovered that people who watched a comedic TV spot instead of a news report or reality television show performed better on cognitive tests following the films. That's not all: humor has also been shown to activate areas of the brain essential for creativity and problem solving.

DECEMBER LAUGHTER: Your Story

I n today's world of heightened hostilities, increased tensions, and more division than we've seen in decades, I believe we need laughter now more than ever before. While you don't have to wear a silly tiara on a daily basis, you will gain incredible mental, emotional, and even physical benefits by striving to bring more laughter into your life any way you can. Here are ten ways to make this month's Laughter Challenge your own and bring more joy and laughter into your life for a healthier, happier you.

1. DISCOVER NEW WAYS TO LAUGH ON A REGULAR BASIS. The goal of this month's challenge is to laugh as much as possible, whenever and in whatever way you can. Before the month begins, spend some time thinking about what makes you laugh and how you can incorporate more time for levity in your life. You don't have to wear a silly tiara, cape, or other item to be successful at this month's challenge. Instead, consider reading the morning comics, watching more funny films or TV shows, or finding a comedian online whom you can stream on a regular basis. Or book a night to attend a stand-up comedy show, follow a few Twitter or Instagram accounts that make you laugh, or even attend a virtual or real-life class of laughter meditation or yoga. This is the time to explore your funny bone.

2. FIND A COMEDY CATALYST IF YOU'D LIKE. If you do want to try using a tangible item like my tiara to help you laugh more this month, it certainly won't impair your progress. If you have

kids, dig around in their toy chests or playrooms for an item like a silly tutu, oversize Nerf gun, or funny-looking stuffed animal that can make you chuckle on sight. If you don't have kids, take a trip to your local dollar store or think about your last Halloween costume party to find a cape, mask, cheap piece of jewelry, pair of glasses, fake nose, headpiece, or other accessory that makes you smile. Don't worry if your comedy catalyst doesn't make you laugh out loud—while ideal, if your catalyst makes you feel good, then it's doing its job. Now keep it in a visible place and use it as often as you can.

3. FORGET ABOUT RULES OR DAILY QUOTAS. The goal of this month is to laugh more, not force yourself to do things you don't want to do. Don't think about how much or how often you're laughing or whether you're successful at this month's challenge. If you remind yourself to bring more levity and joy into your life on a near daily basis, you're nailing this month's challenge.

4. TURN TO LAUGHTER WHEN YOU'RE STRESSED, SAD, ANGRY, OR MIRED IN EVERYDAY LIFE. I discovered this month the tiara worked best—or garnered my biggest belly laughs—when I was feeling stressed, serious, or simply doing something humorless, like getting ready for work or walking my dog. The juxtaposition of laughing out loud when you're down, preoccupied, or simply dealing with "real life" has the biggest potential to overhaul your mood and bring major physical and emotional benefits. Try it by flipping on a funny film, looking at your witty Instagram follows, or picking up a book you know will make you chuckle whenever you're feeling blue or stressed.

5. TRY TO MAKE OTHERS LAUGH. One of the biggest sources of amusement and subsequent satisfaction for me during the

laughter month was using the tiara to try to make my children, friends, and colleagues laugh. Spend time with friends and family during the challenge who make you laugh or with whom you like to joke, play games, or watch funny films and shows you love.

6. REMEMBER YOU'RE DOING SOMETHING CRITICAL FOR YOUR HEALTH. If you're a type A, goal-oriented, or no-nonsense kind of person, you may struggle with the unquantifiable focus of this month's challenge. While it's easy for most to understand the immediate benefits of abstaining from alcohol, taking more steps, or making time for aerobic exercise, setting an intent to laugh more isn't quantitative and your progress or the results aren't as calculable. But laughing, as research shows us, is absolutely critical for our overall physical and emotional health. And usually those serious types who might be dismissive of a laughter challenge are exactly the ones who could benefit most from focusing an entire month on bringing more levity to life.

7. HANG OUT WITH KIDS. There's nothing like being surrounded by children and their natural sense of wonderment to help you smile and laugh. If you have children, spend more time with them in their preferred environment, like a playground, party, or amusement park. If you don't have kids, consider taking a trip with friends to an amusement park, local parade, children's theater, or other activity designed to delight kids, all of which can help you rediscover your inner child and sense of joy.

8. SMILE MORE. When you smile, it activates feel-good chemicals in your brain and helps your mind and body relax, setting you up to be more open, physically and mentally, to laughter and levity. Try starting the day with a smile and

approaching everyone you meet—stranger, colleague, or family member—with a smile on your face. Not only will this make you look more attractive and sincere to the other person, it can help others relax, too, causing a contagious chain of feel-good emotions that will only improve and lift the day for you and those around you.

9. GIVE YOURSELF PERMISSION TO BE SILLY. A critical step for me during my Laughter Challenge was recognizing that it's perfectly okay and even beneficial to take time to be silly, even when (or perhaps especially when) everything else in your life feels serious. Allowing yourself the space and time to be silly builds confidence and self-love and puts you in the right mental and emotional place to let more laughter and levity in.

10. STAY POSITIVE AND DON'T TAKE YOURSELF TOO SERIOUSLY. Keeping a positive attitude and mental perspective during stressful times will go a long way to improving your overall wellness and helping you to become a happier, healthier person, inside and out. We all have problems, but it helps to put them into perspective. If you're not dying or tasked with the chore of curing cancer, you can and will get over your hurdles—and maintaining a positive attitude and not taking your personal, professional, or financial woes too seriously will help you conquer life's challenges while staying healthy and happy.

    We only have one life, after all. And I suggest you live it with the most joy, laughter, and light you can possibly let in.

Turning Challenges into Change

Every challenge I chose to tackle in 2018, I did because it served not only a specific purpose but also had the potential to impact my health and overall well-being in a very meaningful and viable way. I've never been interested in challenging myself simply for challenge's sake. Instead, with each monthly mission, I wanted to learn exactly how and why to make that practice part of my life so that it was not just a temporary focus for thirty days but an ingrained habit for the foreseeable future.

Before I began my mindful year, I had never completed a health or wellness challenge of any kind. At the start of January, I thought I'd simply give up alcohol for thirty days and that'd be it. But by the end of the month, I felt so incredible—and incredibly empowered—that one month turned into two, two led to three, and to this day, I still track how many drinks I consume, writing down each actual serving on my kitchen calendar and making sure I never top seven servings per week.

The same thing happened after every wellness challenge I did during the year. During each month, I disciplined myself to adopt a habit long enough to experience the benefits it brings while learning how to best work that habit into my everyday routine and overall life. As a result, after each month, I knew precisely how and why to continue to make the habit part of my daily or weekly schedule for months to come.

Now that I've finished the full year, there have been many instances when I've combined most, if not all, of my mindful challenges into one single day—waking up to meditate, doing some push-ups and planks before my shower, grabbing my water bottle to hydrate as I head out the door, passing over the carne asada for more vegetables at lunch, checking my step counter, and getting in an after-work jaunt up to SoulCycle for some cardio, et cetera. This process has been intuitive or something that happened organically, not something I've had to remind or force myself to do. In one way, I feel like a winning game-show contestant who can spin a wheel at any time and pick one of my twelve challenges to see if I've done it for the day or whether I want to do it to benefit my body, mind, and mood.

Combining the challenges in aggregate has also given me the feeling that I have more control over my health than I've ever had before. Before my challenge year, I used to worry all the time whether and how to incorporate certain habits into my routine that I knew would make me feel better or were necessary for overall health. Now, though, I feel like I can easily and seamlessly unlock these practices whenever I want, letting them into my life without upsetting my daily routine or mandating amazing amounts of discipline.

If you follow along with me for your own mindful year, I promise you will also learn how to easily and seamlessly turn some, if not all, the challenges into lifelong habits. I encourage you to think of each and every month as an experiment in yourself, giving you the opportunity to explore how to be your best self every day going forward. When you've finished the year, combine what you've discovered about yourself with these twelve best tips and you can and will be able to turn every challenge into lifelong change.

1. USE A WALL CALENDAR TO TRACK YOUR ALCOHOL INTAKE, CARDIO, MEDITATION, STEPS, OR OTHER HABITS: YOUR VISUAL

PROGRESS WILL MOTIVATE YOU TO MAINTAIN. This simple little trick has helped me to sustain so many challenges, especially my dry month, aerobic exercise, and meditation mission. How it works: I keep a big, old-school paper wall calendar in the most visible place in my apartment—my kitchen—and write down the number of drinks I have each week, the days I meditate, and the type and duration of the cardio activity I do. This way, I can quickly add up how many drinks I've had, see how much I've worked out and what exactly I've done, and how long it's been since my last meditation morning. Writing down my behavior in a visible place holds me accountable for all these practices every day, encouraging me to keep these habits going in fear of seeing a blank and bleak calendar.

Why not use the calendar app on my phone? To begin with, you have to remember to open up the app, which means it won't work as a spontaneous visual reminder or motivator. And typing in what I've drunk or done on a small screen doesn't give me the same satisfaction as writing it out in bright pen or checking days off on a big calendar I see every time I walk in or out of my kitchen.

2.   DO IT FIRST THING IN THE MORNING. Over the last year, I learned over and over again that doing something first thing in the morning, whether it's planks and push-ups, meditating, stretching, a cardio workout, or simply getting steps on a hotel treadmill, guarantees me my best chance at success. Taking on health habits in the morning means that if my day gets insanely busy, social or family obligations suddenly arise, or I'm simply too stressed or upset at the end of the day to even consider the idea of habit X, I don't have to worry about it—I've already done what I've wanted to feel strong, healthy, and happy. This isn't just a personal predilection, either: multiple studies show people

who exercise, meditate, or conquer a similar health feat first thing in the morning are more likely to stick with the habit and do it more frequently than those who work out or meditate in the afternoon or evening.

3. SET YOUR ALARM THIRTY TO FORTY-FIVE MINUTES EARLIER EVERY DAY. During my meditation month, I discovered that getting up thirty to forty-five minutes earlier made all the difference between starting my day with positive, focused energy and allowing myself to feel more distracted, anxious, and less connected with myself and the world around me for the rest of the day. After that, when I'd wake up was an obvious choice!

    Meditation isn't the only reason to set your alarm earlier: if you struggle to find time to stretch, work out, do planks and push-ups, go for a walk around the block, or do anything for yourself that makes you feel healthy and happy, I recommend getting up thirty minutes to an hour earlier every day. Don't just take my word: lots of research shows early risers are more proactive, productive, consistent, successful, and even happier than those who try to tackle tasks at night. Studies conducted on the most successful people in the world show they almost always wake up early, not because they necessarily enjoy it, but because they know it will help them accomplish the things that will make them thrive, both personally and professionally.

4. CONSIDER HEALTHY HABITS LIKE EXERCISE AS IMPERATIVE TO YOUR DAY AS BRUSHING YOUR TEETH. I tell my patients to think about exercise like you do brushing your teeth: it's a nonnegotiable part of your day, something you simply have to do for basic health and well-being. The same thinking should apply to habits like hydration, sleep, and eating more vegetables—these practices should be as essential to your

day as taking a shower or getting dressed. You'd likely never leave for work without a shower and the right outfit—by the same token, we shouldn't take on any day without trying to move our bodies, drink enough water, get adequate sleep, and eat some life-sustaining vegetables. While there are always those crazy days when you simply just can't fit in a workout, eight hours of sleep, or any broccoli or spinach, viewing these habits as nonnegotiable components of your day ensures you'll do them often enough so that they become part of your weekly regimen.

5. TELL YOURSELF JUST ONE PUSH-UP, FIFTY STEPS, OR FIVE MINUTES OF CARDIO. I used to think that if I didn't have an hour to work out, it wasn't worth even stepping foot inside a gym. But over the last year, I've learned that you can accomplish a lot with your body in twenty minutes. And I know that doing anything, even five minutes of cardio, is better than doing nothing.

    Whether you don't have the time or simply aren't in the mood to work out, trying to do just five minutes on the treadmill or a bike can have big benefits—and can help turn around your mind and mood, spurring you to work out longer. Similarly, if you don't feel like doing push-ups and planks, tell yourself to do one rep or hold a plank for just ten seconds—again, doing either is better than doing nothing, and you might find yourself eager to crank out more once you're on the floor. The same is true of walking or doing just about any type of physical activity: setting low expectations when you're time-crunched or unmotivated is one of the easiest and most effective ways to get moving and stay moving.

6. FOCUS ON FINDING AMAZING ALTERNATIVES ANYTIME YOU CUT OR REDUCE A FOOD. During my Less Meat, More Plants Challenge and the Less Sugar Challenge, I learned that

it's critical to discover tasty food alternatives so I didn't ob-
sess over the red meat or sugar I was missing. For example, when I stopped eating red meat, I missed it much less
after I discovered smoked salmon with cream cheese and
the Daily Harvest shipments. Similarly, I know I would have
been more successful at my low-sugar mission had I kept
a stash of strawberries with balsamic vinegar on hand for
those times when Jacques Torres cookies suddenly appeared.
Moreover, the process of finding new foods that you enjoy
just as much as the ones you're trying to avoid is a fun process in itself. Just remember to focus on alternatives that
are accessible to you on a daily basis, fit within your budget,
and that you enjoy. Forcing yourself to eat smoked salmon or
cauliflower kimchi when you don't like either, for example,
won't help you be successful and may only make you feel
more deprived.

7.   KEEP REFILLABLE WATER BOTTLES IN YOUR REFRIGERATOR,
     CAR, AND/OR OFFICE. Most Americans are chronically
     dehydrated—and for no reason! This simple tip is so easy
     to do, yet has the potential to impact your overall health
     immensely. To this day, I still keep at least two bottles filled
     with water in my refrigerator so they're always there, star-
     ing me down whenever I open the door and ready for me
     to grab and go or sip from while walking around my home.
     Compared to pouring yourself a glass, refillable water bot-
     tles allow you to quantify your hydration and can motivate
     you to finish a full bottle, upping your water consumption
     significantly.

8.   USE APPS TO TRACK YOUR STEPS, SLEEP, SUGAR INTAKE, HY-
     DRATION, AND/OR MEDITATION. Finding smartphone apps
     to track my sleep and steps was game changing during both
     months, providing the hard data and motivation I needed

to turn those challenges into change. For me, tracking apps are beneficial in two big ways: (1) by providing the real-time information we need to help us adjust our behavior immediately to meet our goals, and (2) by motivating us to work harder when we see data we don't like, and conversely, motivating us to maintain when we see numbers that make us feel good.

9. AVOID PHUBBING, ENJOY PHONE-FREE TIME ON A DAILY BASIS, AND WAIT TO ANSWER EACH TEXT. Maintaining a more mindful approach to technology isn't easy, but I've found it's possible by following some basic rules that are also part of our social decency code. The biggest one: stop phubbing once and for all, or snubbing friends and family by paying more attention to your phone than the people around you during social situations. Not only is this rude, it can and will erode your relationships.

    Second, everyone deserves to enjoy time off the grid every day, even if it's just a few minutes. For this reason, whenever I walk, I still put my phone in my purse. Not only does this give me some precious moments of mental and emotional clarity, it's also immensely safer. If phone-free walks don't apply or appeal to you, consider designating your bedroom as a phone-free zone, which will also help you sleep better, according to studies.

    Finally, I've learned I don't have to respond to each and every text the moment I receive it. Just because someone chooses to send me a text at a certain time doesn't mean the sender requires or even wants an answer immediately. I used to send back knee-jerk answers or hastily typed responses because I wanted to respond even though I was in the middle of doing something else. But now I've learned it encourages better communication and is more respectful to the sender to take my time to answer each text.

10. THINK OF SUGAR AS A DRUG AND TAKE BASICALLY AN ALL-OR-NOTHING APPROACH. During my disastrous Less Sugar Challenge, I learned I can't taste something sweet and stop eating it without herculean amounts of self-discipline. Whether you realize it or not, you're likely similar: powerful research shows sugar acts on our bodies and brains like drugs do, triggering an addictive cycle of highs and lows and cravings and withdrawal that are difficult to resist. In short, the more we have, the more we want. And while a few may be able to follow a three-bite rule around sugar, most of us are better off avoiding processed sweets and desserts altogether, barring special occasions. And remember, I am talking about *added* sugar here.

11. USE VISUAL PROPS TO HELP YOU ADHERE TO YOUR HABITS. I have tons of clothes and accessories in my closet, many that I rotate out seasonally or as styles change. But the one accessory that stays is my bright-orange foam roller, which I keep in my closet specifically to remind me to stretch. Every time I see it, I remember how good stretching feels, which causes me to pull it out on a regular basis. The same is true of my tiara—I still keep it on my kitchen counter or in my bathroom. Just seeing it makes me smile—a benefit I'll take any time of the day—and motivates me to wear it whenever I want or need a good pick-me-up.

12. KEEP LAUGHING. ALWAYS AND FOREVER. If you learn anything from joining me in my mindful journey, I hope it's to look for the joy in life and the miracle that is your body, everywhere, every day, in everything you do. One of the best promises and palliatives for overall health is happiness, which is created from within, not by external factors like money, relationships, or career success. Recognize what your body does, day in and day out—it's an incredible machine—

and have gratitude for where you are within your body, even while you might strive for more. And striving is a cause for joy, too. I promise, there is joy around you, and more important, joy in you. Take the time to find it and celebrate it every day. That's my prescription for wellness, and one I learned this year when I finally started following the saying "Doctor, heal thyself."

Acknowledgments

This book would not exist if it were not for Lisa Sharkey and her amazing team at HarperCollins. Lisa, a former ABC News producer, was the first to hone in on all the ways my January Dry Challenge resonated with *Good Morning America* viewers. Matt Harper and the entire HarperCollins crew have been excited about and engaged in this book since day one.

My colleagues at ABC News recognized the public's massive interest in improving mental, physical, nutritional, and social wellness, and supported both my monthly challenges and this book in a way only the most powerful media company in the world can do. Thank you to Michael Corn, Simone Swink, Roxanna Sherwood, Morgan Zalkin, Alberto Orso, Sandra Aiken, Greg Tufaro, Margaret Pergler, and the entire *GMA* crew. Thanks to Robin Roberts, for always being up for a wellness tweak, and to George Stephanopoulos, Michael Strahan, David Muir, Dan Harris, Cecilia Vega, Rebecca Jarvis, Ginger Zee, Gio Benitez, and Eva Pilgrim for always lending an ear to chat about everything from hydration to meditation. At ABC, I am blessed to work with the best of the best in network news led by James Goldston, Barbara Fedida, Kerry Smith, Terence Noonan, Debra O'Connell, and Julie Townsend, along with her outstanding team in communications. *GMA*'s radio and digital divisions have supported *The Self-Care Solution* from the beginning.

Thank you to Eric Strauss, the head of the medical unit at ABC News. Eric has been the most extraordinary partner I could ask for in helping me deliver medical, nutritional, and wellness information to millions of people. His expertise as a seasoned producer has made his participation in *The Self-Care Solution* invaluable. "Thank you" will never be enough, Eric.

Thank you to my agents at Abrams Artists Agency, Alec Shankman and Mark Turner, and my literary agent and publicist, Heidi Krupp. Those at my medical practice, Hygeia Gynecology, including my practice administrator, Carole Gittleman, my medical assistant, Ana Olivera, and my patients, have always been eager participants in my wellness endeavors. You all have given me tremendous support and encouragement and added fun to these experiments-in-self. Thank you for the professional sisterhood you provide.

This book would not have been born without the amazing writing of my coauthor, Sarah Toland. From the first call, Sarah "got it." As a fellow wellness junkie, Sarah provided not only personal experience but also an inquiring mind to this year-long journey into self-care. Sarah, you are the bomb dot com. Thank you for keeping me on a tight schedule and helping me translate my experiences and ideas into words. I will always laugh when I recall our long conversations often held from our respective cars. The definition of multitaskers to the max!

Thank you to the people who help *care* for me: Lisa Hayes; Deanna Landro; Dora Smagler; Roger Molina and his staff at Allure Salon; Dr. Jeffrey Rapaport; every hair stylist and makeup artist at ABC News; my fitness trainer and owner of PRX, Cliff Randall; SoulCycle; and my friends at Lululemon, APL sneakers, Clean Market NYC, and Mercedes Club fitness center. Thanks to Bob Roth for teaching me transcendental meditation and showing me what meditation can do for my mind.

And finally, thanks to my family. They bear with me every time I gleefully announce my latest health challenge or self-care obsessions. Sometimes they even participate! Thanks to Dr. Mehmet Oz and Lisa Oz for nearly twenty-five years of love and friendship and the perpetual inspiration and motivation to make healthy habits a priority. Todd, thank you for supporting me mentally, physically, intellectually, scientifically, and romantically, and allowing me to inflict these monthly challenges on you and on us as a couple. My children, Alex and Chloe, have not only done these challenges with me, but they have also embarked on their own experiments in self-care, even while being full-time students. Thank you both for letting me teach you the importance of living a holistically healthy life, solidifying little wellness practices from your teenage years onward, and appreciating how important the things we do every day are for our health. My role as your mother has been the greatest gift of my life.

I wish you all good health, joy, fun, and endless curiosity. And I hope you enjoy *The Self-Care Solution.*

About the Author

J ennifer Ashton, M.D., M.S., is the chief medical correspondent for ABC News as well as a board-certified doctor and nutritionist in OB-GYN and obesity medicine. A known and beloved expert in medical health and specifically women's health, Dr. Ashton is a published author, an educator, and a popular television presence. She lives in New York City.

S arah Toland is a writer, editor, and on-air journalist based in New York City. She is the author of several health and wellness books, including the *New York Times* bestselling *Strong Is the New Beautiful* with Lindsey Vonn.